Nurses' Questions/
Women's Questions

American University Studies

Series XXVII
Feminist Studies

Vol. 5

PETER LANG
New York • Washington, D.C./Baltimore
Bern • Frankfurt am Main • Berlin • Vienna • Paris

Susan Rimby Leighow

Nurses' Questions/ Women's Questions

The Impact of the Demographic Revolution and Feminism on United States Working Women, 1946–1986

PETER LANG
New York • Washington, D.C./Baltimore
Bern • Frankfurt am Main • Berlin • Vienna • Paris

Library of Congress Cataloging-in-Publication Data

Leighow, Susan Rimby.
Nurses' questions/women's questions: the impact of the demographic
revolution and feminism on United States working women,
1946–1986 / Susan Rimby Leighow.
p. cm. — (American University studies.
Series XXVII, Feminist studies; vol. 5)
Includes bibliographical references and index.
1. Nursing—Social aspects—United States—History—20th century.
2. Nurses—Employment—Social aspects—United States. 3. Feminism—
United States—History. 4. Married women—Employment—Social aspects—
United States. 5. Nurses—Social conditions—United States—History—
20th century. I. Title. II. Series.
RT86.5.L45   610.73'0973'09045—dc20   94-44165
ISBN 0-8204-2755-1
ISSN 1042-5985

Die Deutsche Bibliothek-CIP-Einheitsaufnahme

Leighow, Susan Rimby:
Nurses' questions/women's questions: the impact of the demographic
revolution and feminism on United States working women, 1946–1986 / Susan
Rimby Leighow. –New York; Washington, D.C./Baltimore; Bern; Frankfurt
am Main; Berlin; Vienna; Paris: Lang.
(American university studies: Ser. 27, Feminist studies; Vol. 5)
ISBN 0-8204-2755-1
NE: American university studies / 27

Cover design by George Lallas.

The paper in this book meets the guidelines for permanence and durability
of the Committee on Production Guidelines for Book Longevity
of the Council of Library Resources.

© 1996 Peter Lang Publishing, Inc., New York

Printed in the United States of America.

Table of Contents

List of Figures

Acknowledgements

One of the pleasures of completing a book is the opportunity to thank those who supported and assisted me. My dissertation advisors, Maurine Weiner Greenwald and Richard J. Oestreicher, have continued to make suggestions and give encouragement. Another dissertation committee member, Jonathon Erlen, has kept me apprised of useful sources. This manuscript is a better book because of their input. My colleagues at Shippensburg University have likewise been supportive of my work. Karen Wagner's thorough review of the manuscript was invaluable.

A number of librarians, archivists, and contact people assisted me. Many thanks to Linda Krit and Eileen Cushey at the Dorothy J. Novello Memorial Libarary in Harrisburg, Pennsylvania; Beryl Gilkes, Peter Preziosi and Dr. Franklin Shaffer at the National League for Nursing headquarters in New York City; Margaret Goostray and Helen Sherwin at Mugar Library, Boston University; Martha Hodges at the Martin P. Catherwood Library, Cornell University; and Edie Ashbury at the Holy Spirit Hospital Library, Camp Hill, Pennsylvania. Kathleen Carlson Mebus, Terry Freed, and Richard Stober, staff members with the Pennsylvania Nurses Association, loaned materials and helped me contact PNA members I wanted to interview. Barbara Christy of Nurses NOW, and Douglas Ednie and Karen Jackson of Pennsylvanians for Human Life and Birthright, respectively, also helped me locate interview subjects.

The staff at Peter Lang Publishing, Inc., particularly Mary McCarthy and Jacqueline Pavlovic provided me with the feedback and support necessary to revise my dissertation. Douglas West of Revelation Design assisted with the preparation of copy.

Several friends helped coordinate the details of juggling archival research, family demands, and a tight budget. Ann Dysktra and Gary Hines, Bill and Jan Hamblen, and Bernard Miller respectively housed me in Pittsburgh, Boston, and Philadelphia. Susan Callan and Kathy Pierich provided childcare during my out-of-town trips.

Most of all I would like to thank my family for their love and encouragement. My husband, John Leighow, shouldered household responsibilities, read drafts, and gave moral support during the arduous processes of research and writing. Our son, John Daniel, graciously shared his mother with a manuscript. My sister, Kathy Williams, and mother-in-law, Janis Leighow, offered the insights only a nurse could give. My parents, Francis and Esther Rimby, encouraged me to both pursue a Ph.D. and write this book, just as they have supported all my other endeavors.

Parts of Chapter 2 were included in *Not June Cleaver: Women and Gender in Postwar America, 1945-1960*, edited by Joanne Meyerowitz. Philadelphia: Temple University Press, 1994.

Introduction

On May 11, 1995 the *New York Times* reported the results of a new Louis Harris survey of contemporary American life. The *Times* article, entitled "Women Are Becoming Equal Providers," noted that forty-eight percent of married women earned half or more of their families' incomes. Wives appeared satisfied with the situation. Two-thirds reported they would continue their employment even if money were no object.[1] The study's results led Colleen Keast, executive director of the Whirlpool Foundation, to conclude that women " 'have firm roots in both the worlds of work and home.' "[2]

Keast hoped this survey would end a long and often bitter discourse about women's work force participation.[3] Public debate about working women was nothing new. Americans had debated the propriety of female employment practically since the first women entered the paid labor force. In recent decades, however, this debate had become increasingly loud and strident, accelerating with each upward movement of the female employment rate. Much of this concern centered on working mothers. Critics predicted that maternal employment spelled doom for both the American family and the larger society. By the 1980s and 1990s fear of societal breakdown had spawned a conservative political resurgence. These conservatives blamed postwar feminism, the 1960s counterculture, and the "Me Decade" of the 1970s for luring women from their rightful place — the home. Rallying around the cry of "family values" the New Right called for a return to traditional gender roles. They looked to the 1950s as a golden era for the American family replete with bread-winning fathers, homemaking mothers, and well-mannered children.

These conservative critics, however, missed two important points. First of all, female employment was not unique to the baby-boom generation. Married women's labor force participation increased steadily throughout the twentieth century.[4] During these same decades fertility dropped and marital dissolution grew. The early marriage, high birth, and lower divorce rates of the 1950s were an aberration. Baby-boomers' behavior was consistent with the patterns established by earlier generations.[5]

Secondly, both New Right conservatives and the larger U.S. public misunderstood the period between the late 1940s and the mid-1960s. As historian Elaine Tyler May argued Americans indeed "rushed to traditional gender roles" after World War II. "Domestic ideology" occupied an important place in a postwar culture concerned with security and protection.[6] But women's roles were also complex. During the so-called golden age of the family, twenty percent of mothers held jobs. The labor force participation of women with school-aged children nearly approached that of those who were childless.[7] A number of trends — increased demand for workers in the service sector, rising wages, attractive working conditions, and postwar consumerism — fueled this movement into the work force.[8] The public discourse was likewise complex. Government agencies, concerned about proper resource utilization, promoted married women's employment.[9] Popular nonfiction publicized and celebrated the achievements of female workers, politicians, and activists.[10]

Yet in a number of ways the years after World War II *were* different. Married women's employment didn't just grow in those years, it erupted. Between 1950 and 1980 their labor force participation rose from 21.6 to 50.1 percent. This increase was three times greater than that of the 1890-1940 period.[11] The employed woman's profile also changed. During the 1950s and early '60s working mothers were typically over thirty-five and had children between the ages of six and seventeen. After the mid-1960s large increases occurred in the labor force participation of younger mothers with preschool children. These younger women were also more likely to be college graduates.[12] Attitudes changed as well. Working women had fought discrimination since the earliest days of the Industrial Revolution.[13] Now their efforts intensified. Work assumed a new importance in women's lives and they were less tolerant of unfairness. By the 1950s the Women's Bureau of the Department of Labor was already flooded with complaints of discrimination.[14] Union women stepped up earlier campaigns for equal pay and fair hiring and promotion practices.[15] By the late 1960s and early 1970s the fight against workplace sexism intensified. Younger women, often college-educated and politically active, joined the effort. Many defined their problems in feminist terms and considered themselves part of the re-emerging women's movement.[16]

These phenonema raise a number of questions for historians. First, why did female wage-earners come to identify so strongly with work roles in the postwar period? Secondly, did all women internalize the role of worker, or was this unique to women from particular age cohorts, occupations, or educational backgrounds? Thirdly, which women responded to feminism and how did they utiilze it to solve their work-related problems? Fourthly, did women workers embrace the entire feminist program or did they accept certain parts and reject others? The conservative backlash against the women's movement during the 1980s raises a final question.[17] Why did women who identified with traditional gender roles find feminism so threatening?

Studying nursing is an excellent way to answer these questions. Postwar employment trends affected nurses as they affected women in other occupations. Expansion of the health care sector, rising wages, increasingly attractive working conditions, and the desire for a middle class life style encouraged nurses to re-enter the work force in the 1950s and early 1960s. By the late 1960s and 1970s nurses, particularly those who were born after 1940, college-educated, and working at elite jobs, intensified earlier efforts to raise salaries and status. As they encountered resistance from male-dominated medicine and health care administration, some R.N.s acquired a feminist consciousness. They believed their problems stemmed directly from the sexual composition of their profession and the social construction of gender roles. They offered critiques of both medicine's dominance of nursing and male supremacy over females.[18] They exhibited a will to reform society and assumed a conviction that change was possible.[19] Feminist nurses adopted those features of the women's movement which spoke to their experiences as women workers. They used feminism to re-define and resolve professional issues in a variety of ways. At the same time more traditional nurses fought to preserve their time-honored roles of wife, mother, and angel of mercy.

In the post-World War II era nursing also became a highly visible, and therefore an easily studied, profession. R.N.s rapidly grew in number and importance as Americans used more health care services. Furthermore, from 1946 to 1986 over ninety percent of registered nurses were female.[20] Since eighty percent of American women work in feminized occupations, nurses' experiences and reactions during the postwar period should be particularly insightful.[21] Finally, nursing reflects patterns present in the larger society. Like American women in general, nurses are divided by education and class. R.N.s have also endured sexism. Although relatively few men entered the field of nursing, historically physicians controlled nurses, particularly those employed in hospitals. Female directors of nursing have traditionally had little autonomy from male medical chiefs of staff and hospital administrators. Their situation parallels that of women in the larger society who have been governed by fathers, husbands, and male bosses.

This study examines a number of events and trends. Chapter 1 describes nursing prior to 1946, providing readers with some historical background on the profession. Chapter 2 traces changes in nurses' labor force participation rates during the early postwar period and analyzes the factors which caused wives and mothers to prolong or reenter paid labor. Expansion of the U.S. health care system and changes within the field of nursing will be given special attention. These phenomena made paid work both acceptable and feasible for the married, child-rearing nurses of the 1950s and '60s. Chapter 3 explores the growth of college attendance among R.N.s and how this experience, particularly during the 1960s, transformed women's self-images, attitudes about work, and perceptions of sexism.

Chapter 4 examines the ways in which both younger college-educated nurses and those in more elite fields discovered and accepted the postwar women's movement. Chapter 5 deals with the myriad ways nurses responded to feminism in the 1970s and 1980s. During these years R.N.s in a wide variety of occupational settings used feminist rhetoric and tactics to combat unacceptable salaries, low status, lack of autonomy, and the difficulties of juggling work and family. Chapter 6 studies the limits of feminism for nursing. The movement's initial insensitivity, negative media coverage, and the conservative resurgence of the 1980s kept feminist nurses from mobilizing more colleagues and promoting wider change. At the same time Chapter 6 examines the complexity of the women's movement's impact. Even nurses who shudder at the term "feminist" have adopted some of the movement's tenets such as equal pay for equal work and egalitarian marriage.

This study proves that many postwar women internalized the roles of wage-earner and professional. They eagerly responded to economic and social forces which facilitated married women's employment and the acquisition of a college education. Some of those who re-identified themselves perceived discrimination in both their work sites and the larger society. They sought redress in a number of ways — the Equal Rights Amendment, the comparable worth movement, reproductive choice — to name a few. The tactics they used were likewise diverse ranging from consciousness raising to lobbying, collective bargaining to litigation. This study also proves, however, that a large segment of female wage-earners rejected feminism. They felt threatened by an ideology which seemed to demean their roles as wives and mothers. The women's movement thus helped fuel the contemporary debate over female employment and family values. As Americans struggle with the persistence of sexism and changing gender roles, we need to understand what postwar women questioned, why they questioned, and why their queries have remained largely unanswered.

Endnotes

1. Tamar Lewin, "Women Are Becoming Equal Providers," *New York Times*, 11 May 1995, sec. 1.

2. Lewin, "Equal Providers."

3. Lewin, "Equal Providers."

4. Claudia Goldin, *Understanding the Gender Gap: An Economic History of American Women* (New York: Oxford University Press, 1990), 17-19; Steven D. McLaughlin et al., *The Changing Lives of American Women* (Chapel Hill: The University of North Carolina Press, 1988), 94.

5. Andrew J. Cherlin, *Marriage, Divorce, Remarriage* (Cambridge, Ma.: Harvard University Press, 1981), 20-22; Goldin, *Understanding the Gender Gap*, 140-141; Elaine Tyler May, *Homeward Bound: American Families in the Cold War Era* (New York: Basic Books, Inc, Publishers, 1988), 3-9; McLaughlin et al., *Changing Lives*, 55, 60, 127.

6. May, *Homeward Bound*, 5-11.

7. Diane Crispell, "Myths of the 1950s," *American Demographics* 14 (August 1992): 42.

8. For an analysis of service sector demand, wages and working conditions see Goldin, *Understanding the Gender Gap*, 174-184; McLaughlin, et al., *Changing Lives*, 98-100. For a discussion of the impact of post World War II consumerism see Kenneth T. Jackson, *Crabgrass Frontier: The Suburbanization of the United States* (New York: Oxford University Press, 1985), 243-244; May, *Homeward Bound*, 165-168.

9. Susan M. Hartmann, "Women's Employment and the Domestic Ideal in the Early Cold War Years," in *Not June Cleaver: Women and Gender in Postwar America, 1945-1960*, ed. Joanne Meyerowitz (Philadelphia: Temple University Press, 1994), 87-94.

10. Joanne Meyerowitz, "Beyond the Feminine Mystique: A Reassessment of Postwar Mass Culture, 1946-1958," in *Not June Cleaver*, 232-241.

11. Goldin, *Understanding the Gender Gap*, 17-19; McLaughlin et al., *Changing Lives*, 93.

12. Cherlin, *Marriage, Divorce, Remarriage*, 50; Crispell, "Myths of the 1950s," 42; Goldin, *Understanding the Gender Gap*, 138-154, 174-184; McLaughlin, et al., *Changing Lives*, 34-35, 92-100.

13. For a discussion of women's protests in the 1820s and 1830s see Alice Kessler-Harris, *Out to Work: A History of Wage-Earning Women in the United States* (New York: Oxford University Press 1982), 40-43.

14. Kessler-Harris, *Out to Work*, 308.

15. Dorothy Sue Cobble, "Recapturing Working Class Feminism: Union Women in the Postwar Era," in *Not June Cleaver*, 61-68.

16. Sara Evans, *Personal Politics: The Roots of Women's Liberation in the Civil Rights Movement and the New Left* (New York: Alfred A. Knopf, 1979), 17-23, 98-101, 159-189, 232; Sylvia Ann Hewlitt, *A Lesser Life: The Myth of Women's Liberation in America* (New York: William Morrow and Company, Inc, 1986), 18-23; Ethel Klein, *Gender Politics: From Consciousness to Mass Politics* (Cambridge, Ma.: Harvard University Press, 1984), 34, 39; Linda J. Waite, "Working Wives: 1940-1960," *American Sociological Review*, 4 (February 1976): 65.

17. For an analysis of 1980s conservatism and its rejection of the women's movement see Hewlitt, *A Lesser Life*, 147, 179-180; Rebecca E. Klatch, *Women of the New Right* (Philadelphia: Temple University Press, 1987), 122-127, 131-139; Kristin Luker, *Abortion and the Politics of Motherhood* (Berkeley: University of California Press, 1984), 194-215; Jane J. Mansbridge, *Why We Lost the ERA* (Chicago: University of Chicago Press, 1986), 5-6, 20, 90-93, 99-104, 108-115.

18. For an analysis of sex discrimination in health care see JoAnn Ashley, "About Power in Nursing," *Nursing Outlook* 21 (October 1973): 637-641; JoAnn Ashley, "Nursing and Early Feminism," *American Journal of Nursing* 75 (September 1975): 1465-1467.

19. I am indebted to Nancy Cott for this definition of feminism. See Nancy F. Cott, "What's in a Name? The Limits of 'Social Feminism,' or, Expanding the Vocabulary of Women's History," *Journal of American History* 76 (December 1989): 825-827.

20. Philip A. Kalisch and Beatrice J. Kalisch, *The Advance of American Nursing*, 2nd ed. (Boston: Little, Brown, and Company, 1986), 645; Sara E. Rix, ed., *The American Woman 1988-89: A Status Report* (New York: W.W. Norton & Company 1988), 382.

21. Feminized occupations are those in which at least seventy-five percent of the practitioners are women. See James W. Grimm, "Women in Female-Dominated Professions," in *Women Working*, ed. Ann H. Stromberg and Shirley Harkess (Palo Alto, Ca.: Mayfield Publishing Company, 1978), 295; Edward Gross, "Plus Ca Change...?" The Sexual Structure of Occupations Over Time," *Social Problems* 16 (Fall 1968): 202.

CHAPTER 1:

"Learning to be Girls:" Nursing Before 1946

The word nurse conjures up a variety of images, the heroic R.N.s in the television series M*A*S*H and China Beach, the domineering head nurse in Ken Kesey's *One Flew Over the Cuckoo's Nest*, the big-bosomed sex symbols featured in countless "get well" greeting cards. Whatever the image, one envisions a woman. Most nurses transcend these stereotypes. Debunking unflattering images has been, in fact, a major focus of nursing groups since the onset of professionalization. Yet, perceiving nurses as women *is* accurate. Throughout American history nursing has traditionally been performed by females. Because it is a woman's occupation, nursing has experienced unique situations and problems unknown in the male-dominated professions.

From the colonial period through the Civil War, women ministered to sick and dying family members, friends, and neighbors in the home. During these years the household served many purposes. It functioned as workshop, school, and infirmary as well as living space. Medical care consisted primarily of administering special diets, applying poultices, and changing dressings. Since these tasks mirrored their other domestic responsibilities, mature women could routinely teach nursing skills to daughters and female servants.[1] Women also performed more public nursing functions such as attending each other in childbirth. Midwives delivered most babies, assisted by the mother-to-be's female friends and relatives. They called physicians only when complications arose.[2] Working class, female, domestic servants labored in the city hospitals and almshouses which serviced the urban poor.[3] Throughout the Revolutionary War women also nursed soldiers in both their homes and military hospitals.[4]

The nineteenth century Industrial Revolution changed the society which had relied so heavily on household production. Work became separated from the home, allowing a sharper delineation of gender roles. Urban families increasingly produced less and bought goods and services from the market. Specialization and technology transformed many fields including health care. In some ways these changes constricted women's activities as healers. Male physicians, for example, displaced midwives, at least among urban, middle class women.[5]

In other ways, however, industrialization solidified, even expanded opportunities for female nurses. Nineteenth century ideology portrayed women as nurturing, selfless, and noble creatures uniquely suited to deal with pain and suffering. Such beliefs reinforced their roles as nurses. Americans came to perceive nursing as both a part of women's sphere and their duty.[6] Wives, daughters, sisters, and servants continued to care for family and household members in the home. Secondly, as female benevolence spread into the larger society, middle class women expanded their nursing activities. The Ladies Benevolent Association of Charleston was a case in point. Established in 1813, the elite white women who joined the LBS visited and provided care to indigent white and free black families. LBS members saw this service as a natural extension of their traditional, womanly role.[7] The prosperity which gave middle class women the leisure time for charity work also enabled them to hire nursing services for their own families. Widows and spinsters, often former domestic servants, functioned as what Susan Reverby refers to as "professed nurses," caring for patients in private households. Of course as cities and their poorer classes grew, so did hospitals. These institutions still employed females to perform domestic and nursing chores, much as they had in an earlier era.[8]

As late as the 1860s these women lacked formal education. By mid-decade, however, several factors led Americans to reconsider nurses' qualifications. The Civil War experience convinced reformers that the nation needed trained attendants. Doctors and hospital trustees also expressed concerns about nurses' character. Hospital workers typically came from the lower social classes while physicians were middle class or above. Eighteenth and early nineteenth century hospitals had been characterized by fierce struggles as nurses asserted their rights as workers. Reformers argued that formal educational programs would attract a better class of women. They saw nurses' training as a way to replace recalcitrant, working class attendants with the properly submissive daughters of the respectable middle class.[9]

In the early 1870s nurses' training programs, modeled after the English Nightingale schools, opened in New York City, Boston, and New Haven. These schools recruited young, white, native-born women from the lower middle and the upper segments of the working classes.[10] The pupils reported to female nursing school teachers and directors, who in turn reported to male physicians and hospital administrators. Nightingale had envisioned a hospital in which nursing superintendents and physicians shared power. This, however, did not occur in American institutions because the training schools were not endowed. Instead the educational program was financed out of the larger hospital budget. This funding situation put nursing directors at the mercy of hospital administrators and trustees. All nurses then, students, teachers, and managers alike, were clearly subordinate. The training school and hospital thus replicated both the structure of the traditional family and the division of labor in the larger society.[11]

The lack of autonomy was clearly problematic. At the time, however, the experiment in nurses' training was considered highly successful. The new educational programs created skilled, efficient, and inexpensive nursing services. Throughout the United States reformers rushed to duplicate this model. By 1900 the nation had 432 nurses' training schools.[12] The hospitals which housed them ranged from small town clinics with a dozen beds to large, urban, prestigious institutions.[13]

Until recently the majority of nurses received their professional educations in these hospital-affiliated schools.[14] These programs provided students with an apprenticeship education. Young women lived within a hospital for a period of a few months to three years. They learned nursing by performing maintenance and domestic chores, and practicing required skills on the institutions' patients. Training school enrollees worked long hours. One study estimated that student nurses in the 1910s labored from seventy to ninety hours per week, while the larger work force averaged sixty hours. The apprenticeship system provided little in the way of formal, theoretical education. Critics charged that hospitals used these women as a source of cheap labor, by staffing the ward with students rather than hiring graduate nurses.[15]

As Susan Reverby has elegantly stated, "The objectives of nurses' training rationalized exploitation of students."[16] Along with technical nursing skills, the training schools emphasized discipline. Students wore military-like uniforms and were organized in rigid ranking systems. Superintendents and instructors rigorously controlled all aspects of pupils' lives. Young women ate, slept, studied, and worked according to the institutions' dictates.[17] Schools scrupulously regulated free time. Like many sister institutions, Pennsylvania Hospital's gatekeeper noted in writing when students left and returned. The director allowed no visitors without her special permission.[18] Administrators dealt severely with rule-breakers. In 1911, for example, Boston City Hospital suspended a young woman for attending a baseball game with a male orderly.[19] This discipline, it was argued, was necessary to insure that nurses had the proper character to perform their missions.

The emphasis on discipline was a direct carry-over from the British model. Nightingale herself had stressed the importance of character and duty. American hospital reformers, who were also the advocates of the training schools, likewise believed in the importance of respectable, self-disciplined, obedient nurses. Educators asserted that teaching these virtues was as important as teaching manual skills. Furthermore, nursing school administrators saw themselves as surrogate parents for their charges, obligated to protect young women's health and morals.[20] This training school socialization had a significant consequence for nursing. Women entered the nursing workforce accustomed to being altruistic and submissive. "As nursing historian Dorothy Sheahan noted, the training school 'was a place where ... women learned to be girls.' "[21] Under these circumstances it was difficult for nursing students to confront the oppression they experienced.[22]

By the twentieth century an alternative to apprenticeship education appeared. The University of Minnesota opened the first collegiate nursing school in 1909. By 1916, sixteen colleges and universities had schools of nursing. A decade later the number had increased to twenty-five. By 1935 the nation had seventy undergraduate programs as well as several graduate nursing schools. The graduate programs in particular were designed to train nursing educators and administrators in hospital economics and scientific management.[23] Yet as late as 1945 only five percent of entry-level nursing students attended colleges.[24] Students' modest financial resources and pervasive hostility kept collegiate enrollments low.[25] Employed nurses defended apprenticeship education. They maintained that it both provided students with valuable practical experience and afforded working women a means of upward mobility. Hospital administrators refused to give up their cheap labor supply. Physicians, fearful that college-educated women would compete with them for patients, argued that universities graduated overly-theoretical, unskilled nurses.[26]

Doctors' criticism had some validity, for most nurses performed work which required physical stamina rather than scientific knowledge. Before the mid-1930s most hospital school graduates worked as caregivers in patients' homes. The private duty nurse worked long hours. When called to take on a case, the nurse knew she would be at the patient's bedside literally twenty-four hours a day, snatching meals and rest intermittently. She often stayed on a case for weeks or months at a time. The still-primitive state of medical knowledge and technology made recuperation from surgery, childbirth, or a communicable disease a complicated process. Women who practiced private duty nursing also had to be ready, often at the spur of the moment, to accept any cases their registries assigned or risk unemployment. As hospital schools proliferated, nurses face intense competition.[27] In 1890 the U.S. contained only thirty-five training schools, however, that number had grown to 1,775 by 1920. During those same years the trained nurse per population ratio grew from 16 nurses for every 100,000 people to 141 per 100,000. Between 1920 and 1930 alone the number of trained nurses doubled, while the national population increased only sixteen percent. At the same time, due to the absence of regulation, hospital school graduates competed with "professed nurses" for jobs. Not surprisingly, a 1928 report, *Nurses, Patients, and Pocketbooks*, observed that even in good times private duty nurses were unemployed about one-third of the year. [28]

As independent contractors, private duty nurses had a degree of independence and autonomy which they'd not had as students.[29] But the private duty nurse also served many masters — patients, families, and physicians. Convalescents expected their nurses to behave as mother substitutes — "forever on call, cheerful, and devoted."[30] Private duty patients, usually of higher social class backgrounds than the caregivers, could be both demanding and condescending. Families assigned nurses additional chores in order to "get their money's worth." Upper and middle class families also failed to see them as trained professionals. In many households a nurse became just another servant, even required to take meals in the kitchen with the domestic help. Physicians also had the power to make nurses' lives pleasant, tolerable, or miserable. Private duty nurses were doctors' subordinates, just as they had been during training school days. In patients' homes, however, they lacked instructors or superintendents to whom they could appeal if an M.D. proved incompetent or issued an incorrect order. Physicians frequently used their power to have nurses dismissed from cases. Many women maintained that doctors blacklisted nurses who displayed too much independence.[31] Yet as long as women trained in hospital schools and hospitals remained the last resort of the poor, the majority of nurses had few alternatives.

Graduates of both the collegiate and the better hospital schools, however, found other opportunities. Spurred on by the Progressive and settlement house movements, municipal funding, and growing concern over diseases like tuberculosis, nurses entered the field of public health during the late nineteenth and early twentieth centuries. Between 1877 and 1909 both private and governmental organizations, primarily in the urban Northeast, established 565 public health agencies.[32] The movement grew more over the next two decades. In 1924, for example, 3,629 organizations employed 11,171 public health nurses. These women worked in a variety of settings — settlement houses, private charities, agencies like the Red Cross and Blue Circle, visiting nurse associations, and schools.[33] Public health nurses visited urban slum families, taught basic sanitation and nutrition, treated school children, and operated well-baby clinics. Here they found employment which paid higher wages, offered more security, and guaranteed more autonomy than private duty work. Physicians found treating the sick to be more lucrative and much of public health practice involved the traditional "women's work" of teaching and child-tending. Thus these nurses faced little outside interference. In many areas they operated under "standing orders" assuming the prerogatives usually associated with medicine.[34]

Good jobs also existed within hospitals. Women who held a diploma from one of the more prestigious schools or had a good relationship with a training school superintendent, worked in hospitals as head nurses or instructors. From such a position an ambitious nurse could herself become a superintendent. Like public health positions, administrative and educational jobs afforded nurses better financial rewards and more security.[35] Yet the higher status positions also had limitations. During the 1930s, as private health care services expanded and more Americans used hospitals, public health agencies cut services. Physicians and social workers took over functions formerly performed by public health nurses. As this transition occurred, they lost much of their autonomy and security.[36] Head nurses, instructors, and superintendents had problems of their own. They worked long hours, were required to live on hospital premises, and often found themselves in power struggles with physicians and male managers.[37]

During the 1930s a new position appeared for training school graduates, that of hospital staff nurse. Several factors helped shape this new trend. Advances in medical technology, Blue Cross financing, and New Deal public works funding made hospitals more accessible and attractive to the upper and middle classes. Depression-era hardship mitigated against the use of private duty nurses. Furthermore, under pressure from both the nursing associations and state governing boards, training programs had reformed some of their worst features. Many smaller hospitals had closed their marginal schools during the 1920s. By the 1930s most were attempting to offer formal coursework and had cut back somewhat on their pupils' work hours. Hospitals, faced with rising demand for their services, a glut of trained nurses, and pressure to reform their schools, began hiring graduates to staff the wards. Unemployed private duty workers usually filled these positions. By 1937, ninety percent of U.S. hospitals used graduates on their staffs. In 1946 only one-quarter of nurses worked in private duty, compared to seventy-five percent in 1930.[38]

Hospital jobs afforded many advantages for nurses. Employees worked steady hours and usually received free room and board, godsends for women impoverished by the Great Depression. Since the institution employed the nurse, she also had some protection from the demands of cantankerous patients and their families. Furthermore, directors of nursing provided a measure of safety against difficult physicians. In the hospital women also enjoyed the fellowship of other nurses.[39]

But not all nurses liked hospital staff work, nor were these jobs trouble-free. Women complained about low wages, split shifts, and hospital paternalism. Heavy patient loads kept nurses from giving quality care. The introduction of subsidiary workers to perform non-nursing duties proved to be a mixed blessing. On the one hand, aides freed nurses from some of the dirty work. On the other, many feared that auxiliary workers would acquire on-the-job skills and someday replace graduate nurses.[40] Despite this reluctance to work in hospitals, general duty remained the only option for many nurses because of the severity of the Depression.

No matter what form nursing took, however, it remained "womanly work" and thus a female occupation. As late as 1940 the U.S. contained only 7,500 male nurses. Potential male recruits faced discrimination. Well into the twentieth century only sixty-seven educational programs accepted men. Physicians objected to working with them because they found women more docile. Female nurses stereotyped male coworkers as homosexuals or alcoholics. Men worked primarily in psychiatric or urological nursing, work which demanded exceptional physical strength or where the presence of a woman might embarrass male patients.[41]

Certain groups of women also dominated nursing. Whites were disproportionately represented. In 1910 and 1920, for example, black women comprised 17.6 and 24.0 percent of the total female population, but remained less than three percent of all trained nurses. Jim Crow in the South and a color bar in the North limited black women's educational and employment opportunities.[42]

Native-born females, as well as those of British and Canadian origin, also dominated. While nursing's elite — public health workers, administrators, and educators — came from the middle class, the majority of nurses had more modest backgrounds.[43] Susan Reverby's study of Boston nurses between 1878-1939 revealed that students came primarily from the families of farmers and skilled artisans.[44] Nancy Tomes reached a similar conclusion. She found that the majority of students entering the Philadelphia Hospital Training School between 1898 and 1909 matriculated from the more affluent segments of the working class.[45]

Nursing was attractive to these women because it provided them with a means of upward mobility. American society now considered nursing to be a respectable occupation for women. Nurses, for the most part, treated middle class patients in clean and respectable surroundings. Their wages, when they worked, compared favorably with the pay rates in clerical employment, factory labor, and even teaching. Because hospital training schools charged no tuition (in fact many paid their students a stipend) women with modest resources could readily secure a nursing education.[46]

As was true of most female wage-earners in the late nineteenth and early twentieth centuries, nurses tended to be single. In response to a 1928 survey, training school superintendents estimated that only nine percent of employed nurses were married. Twenty percent of the nurses, participating in this study, actually signed their questionnaires with the title "Mrs." This figure, however, included widowed, divorced, and separated women, as well as those living with their husbands.[47] Nurses were also young. Compared with other female workers, few nurses were represented in the age groups over forty-five.[48]

Working conditions virtually necessitated that this be the case. Given the demanding nature of the work, private duty nursing was a diffi-

cult job for older women. Irregular hours and lengthy cases made combining marriage, family, and private duty practice virtually impossible.
Those who served as head nurses in hospital wards or as training school
superintendents also were single. The selection process routinely passed
over married women, as well as unmarried females with romantic interests or family aspirations.[49] During the 1930s and 1940s as Americans used hospitals more frequently and graduate nurses more often
worked there, married employees were still uncommon. Hospitals required staff members to live on-site. Nurses complained that the pace
of work was so exhausting, only "young legs" could perform ad-
equately. Supervisiors disliked married workers, complaining that they
had high rates of absenteeism and lacked loyalty to the institution.[50]

Although married nurses mobilized to meet the World War II emergency, attitudes remained basically unchallenged. Both the profession's
leaders and married women themselves stressed that they had come
back to work "to meet a defense need." They did not intend to stay
employed during the postwar period.[51] Furthermore, many nurse-
homemakers refused, despite intense recruitment campaigns, to rejoin
the labor force. The *American Journal of Nursing's* (*AJN*) 1941 study found
that ninety-three percent of inactive women considered themselves
unable to work.[52] Surveys in New York's Nassau and Oneida Coun-
ties, conducted by local Procurement and Assignment Committees,
reported that sixty-four and seventy-four percent of inactive nurses
could not undertake employment. They cited family responsibilities as
their reason.[53] In a society which frowned upon married women's employment, nurses followed cultural norms concerning females' proper
roles.

Societal beliefs about women's roles also created occupational problems. American women, interested in professional jobs, were crowded
into the fields of nursing, teaching, library science, and social work.
This crowding created both intense competition for jobs and depressed
wages.[54] When men and women labored together, unequal pay and
discriminatory promotion practices were the rule. Male supervisors
controlled the work of female teachers, librarians, and social workers.[55]
While nurses faced little if any competition from men, they did suffer
from unemployment and domination by medicine. The general public's
failure to appreciate the trained nurse's skills, as well as competition
from untrained women, exacerbated these problems.[56]

In response to these problems nurses created professional associations. In 1883 nursing school educators formed the American Society

of Superintendents of Training Schools (ASSTS). Three years later many of these same women established the Nurses Associated Alumnae (NAA).[57] Black nurses, excluded from these organizations because of race, formed their own professional society, the National Association of Colored Graduate Nurses (NACGN).[58]

The existence of several different professional organizations made concerted effort and communication more difficult. However, the leadership had deliberate reasons, racism aside, for creating several different groups. The associations had both distinct memberships and specific missions.[59] The ASSTS, later known as the National League for Nursing Education (NLNE), consisted of an elite network of administrators and educators from prominent colleges and hospitals. The NAA, later the American Nurses Association (ANA), recruited graduates of the better training schools. While each organization represented a different constituency, both shared the same basic philosophy. They believed nursing's problems could be solved in part by raising standards. They also hoped to sell American patients and physicians on the virtues of well-trained nurses. These measures, they argued, would raise salaries, improve status, eliminate competition from untrained women, and weed out students unfit for professional work. The NACGN both promoted these goals and fought discrimination.[60]

The professional associations concentrated on different, though complementary, tactics. The ANA lobbied state legislatures for a system of licensure and registration. Under such a system, a state appointed Board of Nurse Examiners defined educational and practice standards, approved schools, administered exams to eligible graduates, and granted licensure to those who passed the test. These nurses were permitted to use the title "Registered Nurse" or "R.N." to distinguish them from untrained practitioners. ANA members assumed that these measures would shut down marginal schools, eliminate the untrained and undertrained, and give nursing control of its own profession. At the same time they hoped licensure would shut off the oversupply of nurses, thus resolving the unemployment problem.[61]

The NLNE, in the meantime, concentrated its efforts on professionalizing the nursing schools. It publicized the results of pertinent studies, notably the Rockefeller Foundation's 1922 Goldmark Report. It also undertook its own survey, *Nurses, Patients, and Pocketbooks*, published in 1928. The NLNE used the data from these reports to advocate that educational programs be lengthened, curricula standardized, and small training schools closed.[62] In 1940 the association created an accrediting committee designed to establish a national educational standard.[63] In these ways the NLNE, like the ANA, hoped to elevate the trained nurse's status, regulate the supply of practitioners, and wrest control from physicians and hospitals.

Licensure and educational reform, however, had limitations. Physicians, unwilling to share control with either boards of nursing or better-educated R.N.s, denounced both proposals. Furthermore, neither the American public nor state governments saw much need for nursing reform. When states passed licensure laws between the 1910s and 1930s, most were permissive rather than mandatory. Untrained and unlicensed women still legally practiced nursing, although they could not use the title "R.N." Early state nursing boards frequently included physician members, an obstacle to the autonomy the professional associations so desperately wanted.[64]

Educational reform did not occur until World War II when concerns about efficiency forced hospitals to upgrade or close their schools.[65] Although frustrated, nursing leaders were unwilling to antagonize the doctors, hospital managers, and public they served.[66]

The elite members of the professional associations also alienated the rank-and-file. The average nurse was ineligible for the NLNE and refused to join the ANA.[67] Separated from the leadership by class background and occupation, the rank-and-file did not share the associations' goals. They believed that reform most benefitted administrators and educators from the prominent schools. Those women, not private and general duty nurses, would, after all, teach the students and sit on the state nursing boards. Graduates from the smaller training schools also feared licensure and educational reform devalued their diplomas and threatened their livelihoods.[68] Concerned with their own wages and working conditions, the rank-and-file looked for alternatives to the ANA.

Traditionally nurses had joined registries and alumnae associations for employment referrals, mutual support, and comradeship. Although registries became less useful as nurses moved into hospital jobs, the alumnae clubs remained strong throughout the twentieth century. By the 1890s the rank-and-file had also formed groups such as the Nurses' Protective Association and the Private Duty Nurses' League. A response to nurses' work problems, these organizations provided information, benevolent services, and a social network for their members. Because private duty nurses lacked time and were physically isolated when they worked, many of these associations were short-lived.[69] During the 1930s, as nurses experienced the Depression and entered hospital work, a few turned to labor organizations. By 1937 both CIO affiliates and independent unions organized them. Those most successful included the Building Service Employees International Union; the American Federation of State, County, and Municipal Employees; and the American Federation of Government Employees. Unionization ocurred mostly in large urban communities in New York, New Jersey, Washington, and California. Nurses who joined worked primarily in public sector hospitals.[70]

ANA and NLNE members, nursing's elite, often middle level managers themselves, opposed unionization. They saw labor organizations as "unprofessional" competitors.[71] Referring to nurses' long tradition of self-sacrifice, the ANA called nurses' unions "as absurd as a mother's union."[72] Although the California Nurses Association organized R.N.s and won a fifteen percent wage increase in 1942, other ANA affiliates rejected collective bargaining.[73] Despite their frustration with low wages and long hours, many rank-and-file nurses also saw unionization as unprofessional, selfish, and unwomanly. As one exclaimed in the early 1940s, "May God save us from that degradation!"[74] Thus nurses largely rejected a tactic which had helped other workers.

Nurses also had mixed reactions to another potentially helpful movement, early twentieth century feminism. Although nurses marched in suffrage parades, no formal links existed between the nursing associations and the women's suffrage groups. Only a handful of nursing leaders — notably Lavinia Dock, Lillian Wald, and Adelaide Nutting — overtly championed feminism.[75] The ANA, in fact, voted against a woman suffrage resolution at its 1908 annual convention. In the 1920s the association, along with other women's groups, refused to endorse the Equal Rights Amendment for fear that it would invalidate protective legislation.[76]

Nursing and feminist organizations failed to unite for a variety of reasons. Some early nursing leaders were conservative and distinctly anti-feminist. They believed women could attain dignity and status within a separate sphere.[77] Others, while more sympathetic, were unwilling to put equal rights before what they saw as the more pressing problems of educational reform and licensure. They supported suffrage to the extent it helped them attain professional goals.[78] The women's movement also rejected nurses to some extent. Early twentieth century feminists disliked nursing's lack of autonomy and domination by medicine. They appeared disinterested in supporting an occupation so closely linked to traditional women's work. Instead, these early feminists preferred to support female colleges and women's entry into male-dominated professions.[79]

Nursing and American society, however, both changed after World War II. The transformation of health care practices, along with wider societal changes, made educational reform more feasible. The increase in college attendance, the civil rights and student movements, and the rebirth of feminism gave willing nurses the philosophy and tools necessary to challenge the medical and hospital hierarchies. Furthermore, nursing itself became transformed after World War II as large numbers of married women permanently re-entered paid labor. Chapter 2 examines this transformation of the nursing labor force and its impact on the profession.

Endnotes

1. Susan M. Reverby, "A Caring Dilemma: Womanhood and Nursing in Historical Perspective." *Nursing Research* 36 (January/February 1987): 5; Susan M. Reverby, *Ordered to Care: The dilemma of American nursing, 1850-1945* (New York: Cambridge University Press, 1987), 1-2, 13-16.

2. Jane B. Donegan, " 'Safe Delivered,' but by Whom? Midwives and Men-Midwives in Early America," in *Women and Health in America*, ed. Judith Walzer Leavitt (Madison: University of Wisconsin Press, 1984), 308-310; Laurel Thatcher Ulrich, *Good Wives: Image and Reality in the Lives of Women in Northern New England, 1650-1750* (New York: Alfred A. Knopf, 1987), 126-138.

3. Reverby, "A Caring Dilemma," 6.

4. Sara M. Evans, *Born for Liberty: A History of Women in America* (New York: The Free Press, 1989), 52.

5. Donegan, " 'Safe Delivered,' " 310-313; Judy Barrett Litoff, *American Midwives: 1860 to the Present* (Westport, Ct.: Greenwood Press, 1978), 139-140.

6. Reverby, "A Caring Dilemma," 6.

7. Karen Buhler-Wilkerson, "Caring in Its 'Proper Place:' Race and Benevolence In Charleston, South Carolina, 1813-1930." *Nursing Research* 41 (January/February 1992): 14-15.

8. Reverby, "A Caring Dilemma," 6; Reverby, *Ordered to Care*, 16-21.

9. Reverby, "A Caring Dilemma," 6-7; Reverby, *Ordered to Care*, 47-48.

10. Reverby, *Ordered to Care*, 47-48.

11. Barbara Melosh, *"The Physician's Hand:" Work Culture and Conflict in American Nursing* (Philadelphia: Temple University Press, 1982), 7; Reverby, "A Caring Dilemma," 7.

12. Kalisch and Kalisch, *Advance of Nursing*, 104-110, 161.

13. Reverby, *Ordered to Care*, 61-63.

14. American Nurses Association, *Facts About Nursing, 1951*, (New York: American Nurses Association, 1951), 51; Kalisch and Kalisch, *Advance of Nursing*, 378, 706.

15. JoAnn Ashley, *Hospitals, Paternalism, and the Role of the Nurse* (New York: Teachers College Press, 1976), 16-52; Melosh, *"The Physician's Hand,"* 41, 47-67; Reverby, *Ordered to Care*, 54, 60-63, 75-76, 190; Nancy Tomes, " 'Little World of Our Own:' The Pennsylvania Hospital Training School for Nurses, 1895-1907," in *Women and Health in America*, 470.

16. Reverby, "A Caring Dilemma," 7.

17. Darlene Clark Hine, *Black Women in White: Racial Conflict and Cooperation in the Nursing Profession, 1890-1950* (Bloomington: Indiana University Press, 1989), 50-56; Melosh, *"The Physician's Hand,"* 50-53; Reverby, *Ordered to Care*, 52-57; Tomes, " 'Little World of Our Own,' " 470.

18. Tomes, " 'Little World of Our Own,' " 470-471.

19. Reverby, *Ordered to Care*, 55.

20. Reverby, "A Caring Dilemma," 7; Reverby, *Ordered to Care*, 52-59; Tomes, " 'Little World of Our Own,' " 471.

21. Reverby, *Ordered to Care*, 58.

22. Reverby, "A Caring Dilemma," 8.

23. Hine, *Black Women in White*, 63; Kalisch and Kalisch, *Advance of Nursing*, 377-379; Reverby, *Ordered to Care*, 149-155.

24. ANA, *Facts 1951*, 41.

25. Kalisch and Kalisch, *Advance of Nursing*, 381-383; Melosh, *"The Physician's Hand,"* 67; Reverby, *Ordered to Care*, 121.

26. Melosh, *"The Physician's Hand,"* 68-74.

27. Melosh, *"The Physician's Hand,"* 85-91; Susan Reverby, " 'Neither for the Drawing Room nor for the Kitchen:' Private Duty Nursing in Boston, 1873-1920," in *Women and Health in America*, 454-457.

28. Melosh, *"The Physician's Hand,"* 86-89; Reverby, "A Caring Dilemma," 7.

29. Reverby, "A Caring Dilemma," 8.

30. Reverby, " 'Neither for the Drawing Room nor for the Kitchen,' " 460.

31. Melosh, *The Physician's Hand,"* 82-87; Reverby, " 'Neither for the Drawing Room nor for the Kitchen,' " 455-457.

32. Karen Buhler-Wilkerson, "Left Carrying the Bag: Experiments in Visiting Nursing, 1877-1909." *Nursing Research* 36 (January/February 1987): 43.

33. In the South, because of Jim Crow, agencies often employed black nurses to serve the needs of the African-American community. During World War I black nurses themselves founded the Blue Circle because the Red Cross refused to hire them. See Buhler-Wilkerson, "Caring in its 'Proper Place,' " 15-18; Hine, *Black Women in White*, 104-107.

34. Hines, *Black Women in White*, 76; Melosh, *"The Physician's Hand,"* 412-418; Reverby, *Ordered to Care*, 109-110.

35. Hine, *Black Women in White*, 64; Reverby, *Ordered to Care*, 67; Tomes, " 'Little World of Our Own,' " 470, 477.

36. Melosh, *"The Physician's Hand,"* 146-150.

37. Tomes, " 'Little World of Our Own,' " 471, 477-478.

38. Ashley, *Hospitals, Paternalism*, 112; Kalisch and Kalisch, *Advance of Nursing*, 498; Melosh, *"The Physician's Hand,"* 160-168; Reverby, *Ordered to Care*, 180-183, 188-191; David Wagner, "The Proletarianization of Nursing in the United States, 1932-1946," *International Journal of Health Services*, 10, no. 2 (1980): 272, 278.

39. Melosh, *"The Physician's Hand,"* 160, 184.

40. Melosh, *"The Physician's Hand,"* 168-180; Reverby, *Ordered to Care*, 188-195; Wagner, "Proletarianization of Nursing," 275-289.

41. Kalisch and Kalisch, *Advance of Nursing*, 626-635.

42. Hine, *Black Women in White*, x-xi, xvi; Melosh, *"The Physician's Hand,"* 111.

43. Melosh, *"The Physician's Hand,"* 10, 123-124; Reverby, *Ordered to Care*, 17, 81; Tomes, " 'Little World of Our Own,' " 473.

44. Reverby, *Ordered to Care*, 79-85.

45. Tomes, " 'Little World of Our Own,' " 473.

46. Hine, *Black Women in White*, xv-xvi; Melosh, *"The Physician's Hand,"* 10; Reverby, *Ordered to Care*, 17-21; Tomes, " 'Little World of Our Own,' " 473-474.

47. May Ayres Burgess, *Nurses, Patients, and Pocketbooks* (New York: Committee on the Grading of Nursing Schools, 1928), 243-244.

48. Reverby, *Ordered to Care*, 111-113.

49. Melosh, *"The Physician's Hand,"* 40-41; Tomes, " 'Little World of Our Own,' " 473, 477.

50. Melosh, *"The Physician's Hand,"* 171-176; A Superintendent of Nurses, "Graduates versus Students," *AJN*, 33 (May 1933): 479-480.

51. Jean S. Alexander, "Letters - Pro And Con," *AJN* 46 (January 1946): 57; Katherine J. Densford, "Letters from Readers," *AJN*, 41 (October 1941): 1203; "Married Student Nurses?," *AJN* 42 (August 1942): 181; Eloise Partridge and Martha B. Teter, "Soldiers' Wives," *AJN*, 43 (June 1943): 567.

52. Pearl McIver, "The National Survey," *AJN* 42 (January 1942): 23-26.

53. "News Here and There," *AJN* 45 (September 1945): 761-762; "News Here and There," *AJN* 45 (October 1945): 861-862.

54. Kessler-Harris, *Out to Work*, 140-141.

55. For a discussion of working conditions in education, library science, and social work see Dee Garrison, *Apostles of Culture: The Public Librarian and American Society, 1875-1920* (New York: Macmillan, 1979); Diane Kravitz, "Sexism in a Woman's Profession," *Social Work* 21 (November 1976): 421-426; Myra H. Strober and Audri Gordon Lanford, "The Feminization of Public School Teaching: Cross-Sectional Analysis, 1850-1880," *Signs* 11 (Winter 1986): 218-220.

56. Melosh, *"The Physician's Hand,"* 88, 91-92; Reverby, *Ordered to Care*, 97.

57. Melosh, *"The Physician's Hand,"* 33-34; Reverby, *Ordered to Care*, 123-124.

58. Hine, *Black Women in White*, 95.

59. Ashley, *Hospitals, Paternalism*, 96-97.

60. Susan Armeny, "Resolute Enthusiasts: The Effort to Professionalize American Nursing, 1880-1915" (Ph.D. diss., University of Missouri-Columbia, 1983), 120, 136, 178-179; Melosh, *"The Physician's Hand,"* 33, 39-40; Hine, *Black Women in White*, 95; Reverby, *Ordered to Care*, 123-128.

61. Armeny, "Resolute Enthusiasts," 391-403; Josephine A. Dolan, *Nursing in Society: A Historical Perspective*, 14th ed. (Philadelphia: W.B. Saunders Company, 1978), 274-275.

62. Armeny, "Resolute Enthusiasts," 163-168; Melosh, *"The Physician's Hand,"* 42-47; Reverby, *Ordered to Care*, 159, 164-176.

63. Ashley, *Hospitals, Paternalism*, 121.

64. Dolan, *Nursing in Society*, 274-275; Reverby, *Ordered to Care*, 126-127.

65. Melosh, *"The Physician's Hand,"* 45-46.

66. Reverby, "A Caring Dilemma," 8.

67. Armeny, "Resolute Enthusiasts," 161-162; Reverby, *Ordered to Care*, 123-124.

68. Melosh, *"The Physician's Hand,"* 39; Reverby, *Ordered to Care*, 131-136.

69. Armeny, "Resolute Enthusiasts," 256-257; Reverby, *Ordered to Care*, 133-135.

70. Reverby, *Ordered to Care*, 197; Wagner, "Proletarianization of Nursing," 283-284.

71. Armeny, "Resolute Enthusiasts," 188; Melosh, *"The Physician's Hand,"* 198; Reverby, *Ordered to Care*, 197-198.

72. Wagner, "Proletarianization of Nursing," 284.

73. Wagner, "Proletarianization of Nursing," 288.

74. Melosh, *"The Physician's Hand,"* 198.

75. Ashley, "Nursing and Early Feminism," 1466; Susan M. Poslusny, "Feminist Friendship: Isabel Hampton Robb, Lavinia Lloyd Dock, and Mary Adelaide Nutting," *Image: Journal of Nursing Scholarship* 21 (Summer 1989): 64-66; Reverby, *Ordered to Care*, 72-73, 130.

76. L.L. Dock, "Letters to the Editor," *AJN* 8 (August 1908): 925-926; Lavinia L. Dock, "Letters to the Editor," *AJN* 24 (July 1924): 834.

77. Ashley, "Nursing and Early Feminism," 1465.

78. For a discussion of suffrage as an umbrella movement which united diverse groups of women see Nancy F. Cott, "Feminist Theory and Feminist Movements: The Past Before Us," in *What Is Feminism?*, eds. Juliet Mitchell and Ann Oakley (New York: Pantheon Books, 1986), 52-54; Nancy F. Cott, *The Grounding of Modern Feminism* (New Haven: Yale University Press, 1987), 29-34.

79. Reverby, *Ordered to Care*, 130.

CHAPTER 2:

"The Most Critical Period Since Scutari:" Nurses' Labor Force Participation in the 1950s and 1960s

In 1955 private duty nurse, Louise Alcott, wrote an article for the *AJN's* series on married R.N.s. Mrs. Alcott described her job enthusiastically. She also took great pains to prove that her house was clean, meals nutritionally balanced, and her son properly supervised. Mrs. Alcott was unwilling to admit that she worked for financial reasons or for personal satisfaction. Instead she insisted that she worked because of the severe shortage of nurses.

> I am sure there are times when I would not feel justified in leaving my home for a big portion of the day if I were doing so solely to satisfy my desire to continue with my career. But my family feels that I am making a worthwhile contribution.[1]

One month later Elinor Quandt, the mother of eight and six year old children echoed a similar line of reasoning. Like Alcott, Quandt downplayed financial and professional reasons for employment and emphasized self-sacrifice. She stated, "My husband and children fully understand the need for nurses."[2]

Louise Alcott and Elinor Quandt were not alone in juggling family and work in the post-World War II era. In many ways they were the next generation of working mothers. Female labor force participation had been increasing throughout the twentieth century. In 1940, for example, 13.8 percent of married women were employed, compared with 5.6 percent in 1900. After World War II, however, this trend accelerated. Although many married women returned to the home during demobilization, 21.6 percent worked in 1950. During the next decade their employment grew forty-two percent. In 1960 and 1970 their labor force participation rates were 30.6 and 39.5 percent, respectively.[3] Mothers, as well as childless women, engaged in paid work. In 1945, twenty-five percent of women with children aged six to seventeen worked outside the home. By 1955 and 1965 the percentages had increased to forty and forty-five percent, respectively. Although mothers of pre-schoolers were less likely to be employed, their labor force participation still rose from eleven to nineteen percent during the 1950s.[4] They significantly increased their rate of employment during the next decade. The ratio of labor force participation for mothers with preschool children to married, childless women was .54 in 1960. In 1970 the ratio was .72.[5]

These trends in female employment seem particularly significant in an era synonymous with domesticity. After two decades of depression and war, Americans seemed eager to embrace traditional gender roles. Marriage rates, which had remained steady between 1900 and 1940, surged after V-E and V-J Days. The marriage rate jumped from 138 per 1,000 unmarried women in 1945 to 199 per 1,000 in 1946. During the 1950s the rate stayed high, between 150 and 167 per 1,000.[6] The median age at first marriage dropped to all-time lows of 22.6 for men and 20.1 for women in 1956.[7] Birth rates, which had also declined earlier in the twentieth century, reached new highs. The total fertility rate during the 1930s had been 2.3. Between 1945 and 1964, the baby boom era, the fertility rate exceeded 3.0. It peaked at 3.7 in 1957.[8] Divorce rates, which had risen to 18 per 1,000 married women in 1945, dropped to 8.9 in 1958 and remained low for the next several years.[9]

A number of factors account for the rise of married women's employment during this period of domesticity. The interplay of these forces created high demand for female workers at a time when young, single women were in short supply. Working conditions, postwar consumption patterns, and demographic trends encouraged the employment of wives and mothers during the 1950s and 1960s.

In some ways, the postwar rush to early marriage and child-bearing actually facilitated married women's employment. After World War II Americans wed at younger ages, had babies soon after, and spaced their children close together.[10] The Kelly Longitudinal Study of 1955, for example, found that eighty percent of its white, middle class respondents had four children within ten years of marriage.[11] American couples, however, did not return to the large families of earlier centuries. Instead, the percentage of women having at least two children climbed from fifty-five percent in the 1930s to eighty-five percent during the baby boom years. Childlessness, which had reached nineteen percent during the depths of the Depression, decreased to eight percent twenty years later.[12] The mean number of children per woman actually declined from 3.3 in 1934 to 1.9 in 1950.[13] Smaller families, early child-bearing, and compressed spacing of offspring, along with increased life expectancy and lengthier school years, freed mothers for work outside the home. Housewives found their family responsiblities lessened while they were still young, healthy, and able to work. Increasing divorce rates also played a role in female employment. After a period of decline, rates began to rise again in the 1960s. By 1962 the rate of divorce had already inched up to 9.4, after reaching a low of 8.9 in 1958. It increased every year thereafter.[14] The upswing in the divorce rate transformed some former homemakers into breadwinners.[15]

At the same time economic, demographic, and social trends, had a signficant impact on both married women's opportunities and their inclination to seek work. After World War II the service sector experienced tremendous growth. Firms particularly needed clerical and retail sales workers. Because of persistent occupational segregation, the labor pool for these jobs was female.[16] Employers had traditionally hired young, single women and persistently discriminated against married ones. But a low Depression-era birth rate, an increase in high school and college attendance, and the postwar rush to the altar significantly decreased the supply and availability of young, single females. The proportion of adult women who were 16 to 24 and unmarried was 15.2 percent in 1940, but only 10.9 percent a decade later. Pressed to fill jobs, employers dropped the marriage bar. As a means of attracting desireable workers, they increased wages and altered work hours to accommodate family responsibilities. In 1940 only eighteen percent of women worked part-time, but thirty-one percent did so in 1970.[17] Organizations such as the National Manpower Council and the Commission on the Education of Women promoted these changes by disseminating information on the positive consequences of hiring older, female workers.[18]

The service sector labor squeeze and removal of the marriage bar occurred at a time when older, married females actually sought outside employment. Some of this motivation came from trends discussed above. Women in their late thirties, forties, and fifties — many of whom had worked prior to marriage — had the time and opportunity to combine paid labor and family life.[19] But the pervasive suburbanization and consumerism of the postwar era also fueled their employment. New suburban housing had mushroomed as wages rose, inflation remained low, and the federal government underwrote construction. By 1947 young couples found it cheaper to buy homes than rent. Suburbia became the place where Americans conspicuously consumed. Along with their ranch-style homes, families also purchased appliances, cars, and household furnishings. Increasingly they spent money on leisure activities and college educations. Between 1947 and 1961 the number of American families rose 28 percent, while consumer spending on households increased 240 percent. Purchases for recreation and automobiles climbed 185 and 205 percent, respectively. Wives' employment facilitated this lifestyle. Their part-time jobs supplemented those of the male bread-winners and enabled couples to buy extra goods and services.[20] It was no coincidence that labor force participation rose fastest among middle class women.[21] Their employment allowed their families to purchase and display the items necessary to insure middle class status.

Historians and social scientists have thoroughly documented the rise in married women's labor force participation and the trends which led to this increase. Much, however, still remains to be learned. Although many factors facilitated female employment, were any more important than others in encouraging women to take jobs? Did the impetus for labor force changes, such as part-time work, come primarily from enlightened and/or desperate employers? Or did women themselves push for change? How did wives and mothers actually feel about their employment? Did they see themselves as merely supplemental wage-earners or did they identify more strongly with their work roles? Finally, what effect, if any, did the employment of married women have on American attitudes about gender?

Nurses are an excellent prism through which to study these issues. The trends in nursing matched those in the larger society. Throughout the 1950s and 1960s, the proportion of married nurses engaged in professional practice grew steadily. The largest increase occurred between 1951 and 1956 (See Figure 1). Married women, who had comprised forty-two percent of employed nurses in 1949, were sixty-four percent of the total in 1966. The majority of these R.N.s, like women in the larger labor force, were older mothers whose children were either in school or in the early years of adulthood (See Figure 2). The median age of employed nurses, which had been 33.9 in 1949, rose to 39.6 in 1962 and 39.8 in 1966.[22] As wives, mothers, and consumers nurses were certainly influenced by postwar demographic factors, economic forces, and social trends such as consumerism.

FIGURE 1: PERCENTAGE OF MARRIED NURSES IN THE LABOR FORCE, 1949-1972[a]

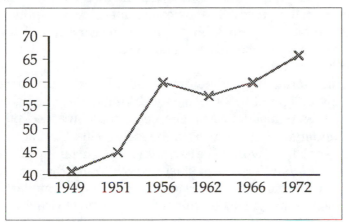

a. *Sources:* ANA, *Facts About Nursing, 1949* (New York: ANA, 1949), 14; ANA, *Facts About Nursing, 1952* (New York: ANA, 1952), 18; ANA, *Facts About Nursing, 1961* (New York: ANA, 1961), 16, 18; ANA, *Facts About Nursing, 1964* (New York: ANA, 1964), 18, 25; ANA, *Facts About Nursing, 1968* (New York: ANA, 1968), 16, 20; ANA, *Facts About Nursing, '74-'75* (Kansas City: ANA, 1975), 6.

FIGURE 2: PERCENTAGE OF ALL EMPLOYED NURSES IN EACH AGE COHORT, 1951-1966[a]

	20-29	30-39	40-49	50-59	60+	Unknown	Total
1951	34	30	19	9	4	4	100
1956	30	25	21	13	7	4	100
1962	25	25	23	18	7	2	100
1966	25	22	24	17	8	4	100

a. *Sources:* ANA, *Facts, 1952,* 17; ANA, *Facts About Nursing, 1962-1963* (New York: ANA, 1963), 15; ANA, *Facts, 1964,* 15; ANA, *Facts, 1968,* 16.

Studying nursing also enables one to focus on the questions discussed above. After World War II changes in American health care triggered a critical nursing shortage. The pressing need for R.N.s, and the solutions to the shortage, were discussed at length in the trade journals and at professional meetings. Articles, reports, and surveys carefully documented the rise in married women's employment and the ways health care institutions recruited and accommodated them. Individual women also wrote, often eloquently, to the nursing press. Here they described their reasons for seeking or avoiding paid labor, their reactions to the changing conditions of work, and their attitudes about job-holding. Studying nurses illuminates the interplay of supply and demand factors affecting female employment, the ways in which women responded to a tight labor market, and the degree to which they identified with work roles.

The transformation of the nursing labor force seems particularly noteworthy in light of R.N.s' behavior during and immediately after World War II. As mentioned in Chapter 1, many married nurses refused to undertake employment in the early 1940s. During demobilization nurses left the work force to resume or begin family life. A study of ex-Army Nurse Corps personnel in 1946 found that one-third of those who left nursing cited marriage as their reason.[23] Similarly, forty-seven percent of civilian nurses under forty planned to leave their jobs, presumably because of family responsibilities.[24] The first ANA Inventory of Registered Professional Nurses, conducted in 1949, found that sixty percent of inactive R.N.s left after 1945. Seventy-one percent of these inactive nurses were under forty years of age and presumably married.[25]

Nursing had experienced an oversupply of practitioners in the 1910s and 1920s. It suffered serious unemployment during the Great Depression.[26] World War II, however, changed this situation dramatically as the military absorbed large numbers of nurses. The war created a shortage for which the profession was unprepared. The 170,599 civilian R.N.s and the 68,000 in the Army and Navy Nurse Corps proved insufficient for the nation's needs. As late as 1944 the ANC and NNC called for 14,000 more nurses.[27]

The shortage did not improve after 1945. In fact, the demand for nurses got considerably higher. The Cold War military build-up, along with the Korean and Vietnam conflicts, led the armed forces to continue recruiting R.N.s. Demographic trends such as longer life expectancy and the baby boom changed the health needs of Americans. During the 1950s and 1960s the U.S. population increased sixteen percent and the proportion of citizens over the age of sixty-five grew twenty-seven percent. In both 1950 and 1960 over half of American households contained children under the age of eighteen.[28] Population growth thus occurred among the very young and the elderly, those most susceptible to illness and in need of preventive care. After World War II the expansion of private insurance provided for the health needs of middle class families. Medicare and Medicaid extended these services to the elderly and poor after 1965.[29] These factors created a tremendous demand for both facilities and personnel as well as the funds to pay for health care.

The tremendous growth in medical research and hospital construction were also major forces in the growth of the health care industry and the demand for nurses. Medical technology and pharmacology had become increasingly sophisticated during World War II. Aided by government investment, medical researchers developed new drugs such as penicillin and sulpha, learned to control the spread of malaria and venereal diseases, and improved surgical techniques. The death rate from disease, which had been 14.1 per 1,000 soldiers during World War I, dropped to .6 per 1,000 during World War II.[30]

Medical research remained a popular cause after the war. Political leaders argued that health care advances were good for public relations purposes and helped the U.S. retain its position as leader of the free world. The public became fascinated with high-tech medicine and convinced that research expenditures contributed to the quality of life in suburbia. Nonprofit and industry groups successfully lobbied Congress for funding. By the 1950s medical research had become a major American industry. In 1941 the U.S. government spent $3 million on research. National expenditures totaled $18 million. By 1951 the totals were $76 million and $181 million, respectively.[31]

Public expectations and medical research fueled a massive hospital construction boom. Americans believed their suburban communities needed hospitals as much as shopping centers and good schools. A public scandal over conditions in state-run mental facilities led to calls for reform, which included newer and more modern mental health centers. In 1946 Congress passed the Hill-Burton Act, which allocated $75 million dollars per year for five years for hospital construction. Congress renewed Hill-Burton many times. Between 1947 and 1971 the federal government spent $3.7 billion for construction. During these years federal monies amounted to thirty percent of all health facility projects and generated $9.1 billion in matching state and local funds. Medical research and public financial support led to the rise of large university medical centers with research, teaching, and clinical facilities. It enabled hospitals to add intensive and cardiac care units in the 1950s and early 1960s. Later in the 1960s newly developed technology and Hill-Burton funds contributed to the growth of nurseries for premature infants, along with respiratory, heart, and neurosurgery units.[32]

By the 1950s health care had become a major U.S. industry. Total expenditures grew from $12.7 billion in 1950 to $71.6 million in 1970. During these two decades the proportion of the Gross National Product spent on health care rose from 4.5 to 7.3 percent. The number of workers climbed from 1.2 to 3.9 billion. Between 1946 and 1960 the number of hospitals increased by 1,182. The existence of beds, availability of new technology, and the assurance of payment led to more frequent use. Patients who had formerly been treated in their homes or in doctors' offices now came to the hospital. Americans increasingly entered and departed the world in medical facilities. In 1935, for example, fifty percent of births and most deaths occurred at home. In both the 1950s and 1960s ninety-seven percent of births and fifty percent of deaths took place in hospitals. The admissions rate of 1960 was double that of 1935.[33]

All of this increased research, construction, and consumption created a massive demand for R.N.s. Hospitals needed them to care for the growing numbers of patients. Other health care facilities also required nurses. Longer life expectancy produced a need for nursing home staff. Public health agencies and schools hired greater numbers of practitioners to care for the home-bound elderly and the baby boomers. Physicians and industrial plants, responding to the demand for health services, also employed more office and occupational health nurses. The demand for R.N.s also triggered a need for educators to train them (See Figure 3).

Nursing leaders, aware of these trends, warned that the wartime shortage would continue, perhaps even grow worse. In 1946 at the ANA convention in Atlantic City, President Katherine J. Densford called for 220,000 more nurses.[34] Over the next few years the *AJN's* editor, Mary Roberts, also alerted R.N.s to the problem. In one editorial she predicted that the shortage would last into the 1960s.[35] In another she compared the postwar nursing shortfall to the challenges Florence Nightingale had faced a century earlier in the Crimea. She called the situation, "the most critical period in the history of nursing since Scutari."[36]

Other health professionals agreed with this assessment. The president-elect of the American Medical Association stated in 1947 that "a serious crisis had developed in the field of nursing." He estimated that the nation had only sixty percent of the R.N.s it needed.[37] In 1965 the Surgeon-General's Consultant Group on Nursing noted that 850,000

FIGURE 3: PERCENTAGE INCREASE OF NURSES
IN NON-HOSPITAL SETTINGS, 1951-1972[a]

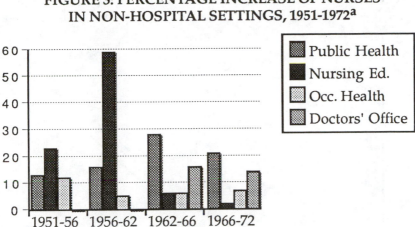

a. *Sources:* ANA, *Facts 1952,* 27, 33; ANA, *Facts About Nursing, 1959*
    (New York; ANA, 1959), 27, 34; ANA, *Facts, 1964,* 9-10; ANA, *Facts,*
    1968, 18; ANA, *Facts About Nursing, '72-'73* (Kansas City: ANA,
    1973), 9; ANA, *Facts, '74-'75,* 19, 27, 31.

more nurses would be necessary in 1970. To accomplish this, nursing
needed to increase its numbers by 8.2 percent per year.[38]

Shortages were particularly severe in several specialities. In 1958
eleven percent of full-time hospital positions remained vacant. As late
as 1967 the American Hospital Association, the ANA, and the United
States Public Health Service estimated that hospitals needed 80,000 more
R.N.s.[39] In 1959 and 1961, according to National League for Nursing
surveys, four and five percent vacancy rates existed in the field of public health.[40] The number of nursing faculty produced annually was only
half of what was needed.[41] The armed forces never seemed to fill their
quotas. ANC and NNC personnel called for several hundred more R.N.s
annually. By 1964 the *AJN* referred to the military nursing shortage as
"acute."[42] This situation developed even though nurse-patient ratios
increased throughout the postwar period (See Figure 4). During these
years both the total number of R.N.s in the United States and the percentage who practiced professionally also grew (See Figure 5). The shortage was clearly due then to the transformation of American health care.

Nursing leaders proposed several different means of easing the
shortage. They called for improved wages and working conditions as
a means of retaining personnel. They also tried to recruit more female
high school graduates, provide scholarships for needy nursing students,

FIGURE 4: RATIO OF R.N.S TO U.S. POPULATION, 1945-1975[a]
(Number of R.N.s to 10,000 People)

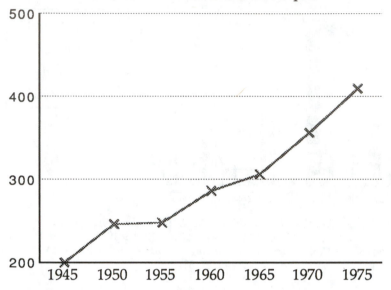

a. *Sources:* ANA, *Facts, '72-'73*, 8; ANA, *Facts, '74-'75*, 4; "Continuing Shortage," 8; Lucile Petry Leone, "People, Nurses, and Students," *AJN* 55 (August 1955): 933.

FIGURE 5: REGISTERED NURSE SUPPLY, 1949-1966[a]

	1949	1951	1956	1962	1966
Total R.N.s	506,050	556,617	650,014	847,531	909,131
Percentage Employed	59.4	60.1	66.7	65.3	67.5

a. *Source:* "Inventory Shows 75 Percent of Nation's Nurses Work," *AJN* 80 (November 1980): 1948.

and develop ways of utilizing staff more efficiently.[43] These tactics alone, however, did not produce enough R.N.s. Dissatisfaction with salaries was not the major reason for the shortage. Only ten percent of women who left the profession took non-nursing jobs.[44] And while the absolute number of student nurse enrollments rose, the percentage of female high school graduates entering the profession dropped from seven to five percent during the mid-1950s.[45] Given the demand for health care services and nurses, the leadership realized that educating more high school graduates simply would not fill the need.[46] The professional associations, therefore, looked to the ranks of inactive nurses. Women who had left nursing to raise children could be tapped to alleviate the shortage. Nursing leaders argued that older R.N.s could provide a more stable labor force than new graduates who would likely marry, get pregnant, and leave the profession.[47] Furthermore, they maintained, married women and mothers could return to work without sacrificing family life. Hospitals had eliminated the practice of "living in" during the 1940s.[48] Jobs in nursing education, schools, and public health agencies were tailor-made for mothers since nurses employed in these settings did not work rotating shifts, weekends, or holidays.

The leadership knew that utilizing inactive nurses was problematic. World War II had proven that nurse-homemakers often resisted paid labor even in the face of a national crisis. Tradition and employer preferences discouraged older, married women from returning to work. In spite of these obstacles nursing sucessfully made the transition from a single to a married woman's profession during the 1950s and 1960s. Between 1951 and 1972 the percentage of married, employed R.N.s increased twenty-five percent (See Figure 1). Forty-seven percent of practicing nurses had been married in 1951. Fifty-five percent were four years later. By 1966 married women comprised sixty-four percent of employed nurses. They made up slightly more than two-thirds of all practitioners in 1972.[49]

This transition occurred for several reasons. The professional associations launched campaigns designed to convince employers to hire inactive nurses and motivate women to work. At the same time desperate health care agencies dropped the marriage bar. They made paid labor more attractive to wives and mothers who previously found nursing incompatible with family life. As a means of securing workers, employers instituted part-time hours, increased salaries, offered refresher courses, and established on-site childcare centers.

The professional associations sought to allay fears about older nurses' job performance and impress the women with the desperate need for their services. In 1949, for example, Mary Roberts asked, "Are we overlooking an important supply when we pass by the group of inactive professional registered nurses?" Decrying this waste of untapped workers she reminded her audience that, "the education of the nurse ... is an expense not only to the school but to society as well." She admonished nurses to remember that a "married woman does not completely escape her obligation to participate."[50] Another nurse, writing in the NLN's (formerly the NLNE) journal, *Nursing Outlook,* in 1953 pointed out that inactive R.N.s made excellent employees. She cited studies which commented favorably on older women's health, intelligence, and emotional stability. She further advised employers to remember that these women "were not so likely to leave the profession for a few years as were new graduates."[51]

These efforts to promote older women as employees continued into the next decade. In 1964 *Nursing Outlook* ran an article entitled "The Aging Nurse." Here assistant editor, Suzanne Friedman, argued that inactive nurses had "years of valuable experience" to offer employers and were "likely to produce superior work."[52] Six years later a director of nursing concurred. In her opinion nurse-homemakers had "insight, depth of understanding, and increased ability to relate to patients and personnel." They made excellent head nurses and supervisors because they had "the knack for getting things done." Furthermore, after a few years sabbatical, the returning nurse brought "curiosity and fresh vision" to the job.[53]

By itself, however, the ANA/NLN campaign could not entice married women back into the workforce. Inactive nurses in the late 1940s and early 1950s found more obstacles than benefits to employment. Despite a desire to resume nursing, inactive R.N.s were dissatisfied with existing employment conditions. Mothers expressed an unwillingness to leave their children for full-time jobs or with unqualified care-givers. As one homemaker remarked in 1947, "Few can leave the house at 6:00 A.M., leaving the children to fend for themselves and a husband to prepare breakfast and get the children off to school. It just won't work."[54] Women complained that salaries barely covered work-related expenses. One New York mother voiced the following concerns in 1952.

> I would like to do some work to keep up with the current trends in nursing. But we have a two-year-old son, and with the local baby-sitters asking $4 a day or more and the hospitals paying nurses $10 a day, it would hardly be worth while. [55]

Inactive nurses also needed more than moral support and verbal encouragement to resume professional practice. Older women were unfamiliar with the new technology and thus had difficulty re-entering nursing. A housewife from Philadelphia wrote to *The Pennsylvania Nurse* in 1953 explaining the obstacles she faced after a five year absence.

> I was petrified at the thought of returning. No one bothered to brief me or
> explain new procedures. I was so disgusted when I finished that tour I have
> been inactive since! I felt that my nursing is gone forever.... If in five years I
> can become this stale, what will it be like when the children are older?[56]

The severity of the postwar shortage forced employers and nursing associations to address these concerns. As the shortage worsened
hospitals in particular found themselves forced to make changes in
staffing patterns. The use of licensed practical nurses and the establishment of two year associate degree programs were partial solutions.[57]
Institutions also implemented part-time scheduling for R.N.s who so
desired. Minneapolis General Hospital, one of the first to experiment
with part-time workers, recruited wives of area G.I. college students.
The hospital allowed nurses who had children, or were attending college themselves, to work as many hours as they chose. Mothers who
wanted to only work weekends, when their husbands were home, received encouragement to do so. The assistant director of nursing found
these new employees "capable" despite their "irregular" schedules.
She therefore described the experiment as a "success."[58]

Other admistrators also found married nurses eager to work when
they could choose partial shifts or weekend employment. Four directors of nursing from Texas, Minnesota, and Illinois, writing for the *AJN*
in 1953, reported that thirty-four to eighty percent of their R.N.s had
husbands and children. All four expressed complete satisfaction with
the women's work performances. They maintained, furthermore, that
married workers exhibited lower absenteeism and turnover than their
single colleagues.[59] Nurses also liked part-time work. One woman, in
a 1966 letter, reported "great psychic satisfaction" from her part-time,
hospital job.[60] Another described the benefits of working two weekends a month. She never needed a baby-sitter and she continued nursing while her husband cared for the children.[61]

Other health care institutions also utilized part-time nurses. During the 1950s civil defense agencies hired married women to teach
classes in disaster nursing.[62] In New York City the director of the Bureau of Public Health Nursing made a conscious effort during the 1960s
to seek out mothers to work in the city's schools. Two years after initiating this program the city had hired 136 additional nurses.[63] Tulsa,
Oklahoma recruited inactive R.N.s to teach Red Cross home nursing
classses, immunize schoolchildren, and screen senior citizens for glau-
coma.[64] Nurses themselves eagerly sought these non-hospital jobs. A
Georgia nurse, discussing her successful return to work in the 1960s,

advised married women to steer clear of hospitals where some administrators still expected R.N.s to work rotating shifts. Instead she urged her inactive colleagues to apply to "birth control clinics, baby clinics, psychiatric daycare clinics, visiting nurse associations, public health agencies, the American Red Cross...."[65]

Because of these successful experiences the number of nurses working part-time climbed steadily upward. Between 1956, when the ANA first published statistics on part-time employment, and 1962, the number of nurses working on this basis increased from ten to twenty-one percent. By 1962 part-timers worked in eighty percent of nonfederal U.S. hospitals and delivered one-fifth of the nursing care received there. Ninety percent of these women were married and eighty percent had children. Their family obligations had made full-time work difficult if not impossible.[66] In 1966 one-quarter of all employed R.N.s worked part-time.[67]

Low wages, as well as inconvenient hours, were initially obstacles to married women's employment. In the 1940s nurses' salaries and benefits had not kept pace with the cost of living. The 1950 U.S. Census noted that R.N.s earned less annually than female teachers, librarians, and social workers with comparable levels of education and job responsibility. They were also among the lowest paid professional and technical hospital employees. Only x-ray and medical technicians earned less than registered nurses.[68] Under the circumstances mothers were reluctant to take on nursing jobs. Wages and benefits increased, however, as health care agencies tried to recruit and retain R.N.s. The growth of medical insurance facilitated this by enabling institutions to pass salary costs along to third party payers.[69] ANA surveys, conducted in 1954 and 1959, found significant gains. Hospital staff nurses' wages increased 24.5 percent, head nurses' salaries rose 18.5 percent, and supervisors and directors made gains of 20.0 and 21.4 percent, respectively. The salaries of public health nurses increased 10.8 and 27.1 percent and those of occupational health nurses rose anywhere from 35.2 to 61.0 percent, depending upon educational levels and position. Nursing faculty also benefitted from rising wages. They received increases of thirteen percent between 1956 and 1958 alone.[70] Nursing leaders still maintained the increases were "not in keeping with their [nurses'] educational requirements and professional responsibilities." Nevertheless, they acknowledged that salaries had "come a long way since 1946."[71]

The trend towards higher wages continued during the next decade. Between 1959 and 1961 median salary increases ranged from 6.0

to 14.0 percent for hospital-employed R.N.s, 19.4 to 21.7 percent for public health nurses, and 22.0 to 30.0 percent for nursing faculty.[72] Wages rose again between 1961 and 1963. Hospital staff and nursing faculty reported the largest gains, 20.0 and 25.5 percent, respectively.[73] From 1966 to 1969 nurses again made "impressive salary gains" as employers passed increases along to Medicare and Medicaid.[74] Hospital general duty, head nurses, and those employed in public heath experienced the largest increases — 39.6, 40.9, and 46.0 percent, respectively. Other nurses, however, also fared well. Hospital supervisors and directors of nursing received raises of 37.0 and 32.0 percent. Occupational health salaries rose 39.0 percent and nurse educators experienced increases of 37.0 percent.[75] Nurses also made gains in paid vacation days, health insurance, and retirement benefits during the 1960s.[76] These salary and benefit increases were a boon to inactive nurses who had wanted to work, but had been discouraged earlier by depressed wages.

For older nurses, however, favorable hours and wages alone were not sufficient inducements. Health care changed dramatically between World War II and the late 1960s. Women who had left the profession were not acquainted with recent advances in nursing and fearful about resuming active duty. Mindful of this situation ANA and NLN state affiliates introduced refresher courses during the late 1940s and 1950s. By the 1960s federal money from the Manpower Development and Training Act and the U.S. Public Health Service also funded these programs. Hospitals and state employment services ran classes as well.[77] Typically refresher courses lasted several weeks. Designed to teach new procedures and bolster women's self-confidence, they combined formal study with supervised clinical practice.[78]

Large numbers of R.N.s both completed course requirements and returned to paid employment. A 1962 study of Chicago nurses, who had taken classes between 1957 and 1961, found that seventy-five percent resumed nursing. Forty-four percent worked full-time.[79] An Ohio survey of refresher course graduates between 1964 and 1968 reported that eighty-two percent of the sample had returned to paid labor.[80]

Refresher students, usually women in their forties and fifties, had not worked for anywhere from ten to thirty years. They understandably felt intimidated by the new drugs, treatments, and procedures they encountered.[81] After completing their courses, inactive women felt self-confident and eager to practice newly-learned skills. One nurse, who completed refresher classes in the early 1960s, enthusiastically described the program's benefits.

I was invited to work in a new hospital during the last week of the refresher course, and I have been there ever since. I found the adjustment an easy one to make because the refresher course not only had prepared me for modern staff nursing, but also had given me confidence in my ability to do good nursing.[82]

Refresher courses helped older nurses return to work. They did not, however, solve the problems of younger R.N.s. Mothers worried about the "present needs of their children," "the well-being of the younger generation," and "leaving children without proper supervision."[83] The twenty-three percent of the Chicago women, who did not return to work after taking refresher courses, cited lack of daycare as the obstacle to their employment.[84] Similarly inactive R.N.s, responding to a U.S. Public Health Service questionnaire, listed the inability to make suitable childcare arrangements as their second most important reason for remaining at home.[85] Once again professional associations and employers found solutions because of the pressing need for nurses.

In the 1950s ANA state affiliates proposed that employers offer maternity leave to pregnant nurses. The associations favored a six to eight week leave of absence, beginning in the second or third trimester and continuing until the infant was several months old. A few health care agencies began to include this in their fringe benefit packages. Nursing directors, writing in the professional press, stated firmly that pregnant women and new mothers should be home. They argued, however, that the shortage made maternity policies necessary. While actual periods of leave varied greatly and pregnant nurses received no salaries during their absences, agencies did guarantee their jobs. Many allowed new mothers to work on a part-time basis.[86]

Agencies which offered maternity leave found it beneficial. A nursing director in 1963 admitted that pregnant nurses caused "headaches." At the same time, she affirmed, she "couldn't run the hospital without them."[87] Public health supervisors, reporting to the *AJN*, believed maternity leave was "a great convenience" for their agencies and resulted in satisfied employees who returned to work "well and happy."[88]

Other employers helped mothers with childcare. A director of nursing at a Kansas hospital, for example, solved her staffing problems by finding babysitters for R.N.s' children.[89] Other agencies reduced vacancies and turnover by providing on-site daycare. Their experiences were similar to those of a New Jersey hospital which, in the early 1950s, had found it impossible to staff adequate numbers of nurses. The enterprising administrator reasoned that married women might return to work if they could find reliable childcare at a reasonable cost. He established a Nurses' Day Nursery which eventually cared for the children of twenty-seven R.N.s who worked the day shift. Housed in a former nursing school classroom, the center cared for eight to twenty-four children, ages five months to five years. Since mothers paid only a minimal fee, the nursery operated at a deficit. The director, however, argued that the added expense to the hospital was "negligible." From his point of view providing the service was clearly worth the expense. Two and one-half years after opening the nursery, staffing pressures were relieved, vacant rooms filled, and patients received more hours of professional nursing care.[90]

Other institutions used similar types of daycare programs. Some offered the service without charge, others provided care for the children of evening and night shift personnel. In all facilities the basic features remained the same. Nurses left their youngsters in safe, attractive quarters on the hospital premises where they played, ate, and napped under the supervision of reliable caretakers. In all the cases reported in the professional press, the nursing labor force stabilized after agencies opened childcare centers.[91] One Tennessee nursing director estimated that without the daycare program, two-thirds of her nurse-mothers would be unavailable.[92] Of course R.N.s themselves were highly supportive. On-site childcare made employment more convenient and alleviated anxieties about leaving young children. Pauline Stack Cooper, for example, warmly endorsed her hospital's day nursery in a 1959 article. The mother of four children under eight years of age, Mrs. Cooper liked having her family nearby. She felt relieved that the youngsters were "just a step away from the wards" and that she could "look in on them" during her lunch hour.[93]

Encouraged by the experiences of the daycare pioneers, more institutions established on-site childcare toward the end of the 1960s. A 1968 Department of Labor survey of 2,000 hospitals found that three-quarters either offered daycare, were planning a center, or investigating the concept's feasibility. Administrators believed the service enabled nurses to work full shifts, stabilized turnover, and reduced absenteeism. The Department of Labor summarized its findings by stating that on-site childcare "tapped the reservoir of women who want to work, but are not free to work."[94]

Part-time work, higher wages, refresher courses, and daycare services facilitated the employment of married nurses who were already motivated to work. R.N.s had a variety of reasons for re-entering the labor force during the 1950s and 1960s. Like other employed wives, they welcomed the opportunity to raise family living standards. Sociologist Everett Hughes argued in the mid-1950s that nurses worked because their "earnings were indispensable."[95] A 1962 Michigan survey similarly found that forty-four percent of married hospital nurses worked solely to supplement family income.[96] An Ohio researcher concluded in 1968 that "helping children through college" motivated many mothers to return to nursing.[97]

Nurses, however, also displayed obligation and commitment to the profession. The hospital training school had thoroughly socialized them to the role of nurse.[98] During interviews with retired R.N.s, historian Barbara Melosh observed that even long-term homemakers still saw themselves as nurses.[99] Everett Hughes found that eighty percent of his sample, even those who planned to have children, had strong career identification.[100] Nurse-researcher Susan Gortner described similar attitudes among senior nursing students in the early 1960s.[101] *Nursing Outlook's* 1962 survey indicated that fifty-three percent of inactive nurses planned to re-enter the work force. The editor remarked,

> Something in nursing is uniquely appealing to those who enter this profession, and such women never really leave it.
>
> We suspect that such persons may find that other activities, particularly those of maintaining a home and family, can never fully use up the store of caring and wanting to help with which they are endowed.[102]

The rank-and-file agreed echoed this assessment. A returning Colorado nurse stated in 1952, "It is the feeling we all have about our work, once we have been in active nursing — the idea of service to others — that draws us back into it."[103] In the same article a Minnesota woman expressed this sentiment, "After the death of my husband, and our three sons went into the armed services, I desperately needed something to do."[104] These statements may well in part have been attempts to staunch criticisms of working mothers. Altruism, particularly in the face of the shortage, was an acceptable reason for employment. But not all nurses defined their motives for working in terms of duty. Others described the intellectual stimulation they received from nursing. In 1947 one wife admitted that full-time homemaking had bored her. She disliked "puttering around in a little two or three-room apartment, wishing I had more to do."[105] A Washington nurse, writing in 1953, listed the following reasons for working, "because I like to keep up with the times [nursing technology], because I like working."[106]

By the mid-1960s, re-entering paid labor was so common, that young nurse-homemakers developed strategies to facilitate their eventual return. In some communities inactive R.N.s formed study groups as a means of keeping up-to-date.[107] One homemaker, writing in the *AJN* in 1965, paid ANA dues, attended local meetings, and read a variety of professional journals. As she explained,

> Through the organization [ANA] I can keep up with the thinking and planning in nursing....Subscribing to nursing publications also helps me keep abreast of current trends in nursing and helps financially support nursing research and literature....

> The next time someone asks me if I used to be a nurse I shall firmly reply, "Yes I *am* [italics hers] a nurse, and I work at it, too."[108]

At the same time, however, women felt compelled to publicly defend their behavior and their mothering skills. One hospital relief nurse had been accused of rejecting her children She wrote the following defense in 1964, "Someone may get the idea that we don't like being home with our families. Quite the contrary."[109] Others, like Louise Alcott and Elinor Quandt, used the personnel squeeze to justify their employment. One R.N., writing in 1966, argued that "the ever-increasing shortage of nurses today" prompted mothers' employment.[110] Three years later another used the same reasoning, noting that the shortage drove "conscientious mothers" to work.[111]

Even nurses with advanced degrees and prestigious positions rationalized their actions. A 1968 *AJN* article — penned by two R.N.s who held masters degrees, were Yale psychiatric nursing instructors, and had three pre-school children apiece — was a case in point. The authors had written advice for other young women seeking to juggle employment with family responsibilities. Along with practical tips, they took great pains to prove their competence as parents. They pointed out, "In many ways, our jobs as mothers are enhanced by our work as psychiatric nurses." They emphasized their dedication to family, maintaining, "We devote as much and sometimes more time to enjoying our husbands and children than we might if we were constantly at home during the week." Finally, they cautioned other women to "consider their husbands' needs" and periodically "re-evaluate continuing to work in nursing."[112]

Even nurses with teenage or adult children described their employment in terms that did not challenge conventional notions about women's roles. One R.N., who returned to work in 1968, perceived a job as "good therapy" for those suffering from empty nest syndrome.

She advised fellow nurses, however, to seek their husbands' approval before re-entering the work force.[113] Another referred to her employment as "a pleasant addition to our lives" rather than as an on-going, professional pursuit.[114] Even the family members who benefitted from a nurse's paid labor often regarded her job as a marginal enterprise. Husbands and children assumed the employed wife would still provide the same quality of homemaking services. A 1969 article, written by Elizabeth Worley, the mother of several teenagers, revealed the difficulties faced by returning nurses, expected to juggle work and family. A refresher course student, Mrs. Worley described her average day in this fashion.

> After spending the day trying to bridge the gap between the flaxseed poultice and Flaxedil, I would rush home to cope with the undone duties of my menage.

> Later, the household bedded down, I tried to concentrate on the brain-boggling reading assignments the instructor felt would be helpful. And I wondered why I couldn't read more than a page without falling asleep.[115]

The transformation of nursing from a single to a married woman's profession, therefore, did not lead to a similar realignment of beliefs about gender. Employer and societal acceptance of working wives and mothers occurred because of a critical nursing shortage. Changes in the work place, such as part-time jobs, allowed nurses to undertake employment without challenging the primacy of their family roles. On-site child care and refresher courses presumed mothers bore the brunt of child-rearing and would not work until home responsibilities lessened. No matter what nurses' feelings were on the matter, health care agencies, U.S. society, and even the professional associations saw wives and mothers as marginal workers. Study after study portrayed married R.N.s as supplemental wage-earners who "helped out" their husbands.[116]

Focusing on nurses, however, does explain much about married women's employment after World War II. The postwar personnel crunch proved to be a key factor in facilitating their re-entry into the work force. Desperate health care agencies raised wages and made accommodations. Employment became both attractive and feasible. Married nurses already had financial and personal reasons to work. As their letters in the professional press revealed, however, they would shun paid labor unless employers removed obstacles. Inactive women indicated that they would not return until the nursing work environment changed.

Once re-employed, married nurses displayed great enthusiasm about their jobs. They took satisfaction in practicing the skills learned in training schools and refresher courses. They expressed pride in their ability to help resolve the nursing shortage and give good care. R.N.s received a sense of accomplishment and intellectual satisfaction from their employment. At the same time they acknowledged prevailing beliefs about gender. Nurses' public statements reflected the social tension generated by married women's employment. Time and again, they referred to the shortage, noting that the needs of the sick took precedence over their own family obligations. The entry of married women and mothers into the nursing labor force did not change attitudes about women's roles. Many nurses themselves saw their employment as supplemental, secondary to their roles as wives and mothers. Employer accommodations recognized, rather than challenged, these traditional beliefs.

Nevertheless, nursing was transformed by the re-entry of married women during the 1950s and 1960s. Nursing's composition changed radically. In 1966, when married women represented nearly two-thirds of all practitioners, a revolution of sorts had been accomplished.[117] Furthermore, the suggestion that married R.N.s had an obligation to work during the shortage somewhat undermined family claims. The wives and mothers of the 1950s and 1960s also had an impact on the next generation. Older married nurses served as role models to the baby boomers of the 1970s and 1980s. Many younger women entered the profession determined to work continuously. This desire came, in part, from the knowledge that an earlier group had done just that.[118] And as married nurses spent more time in the work force, at least a minority tried to maximize their earnings and enhance their status. The growth of graduate nursing education between the 1950s and the 1980s was one manifestation of this desire. Rising enrollments were directly tied to the career desires of professionally-minded married women who re-entered the work force after World War II.

As nurses attended college, particularly during the years of student activism in the late 1960s and early 1970s, they altered many of their beliefs. They re-examined women's roles and nursing's position in the American health care system. College attendance fostered a new career commitment among both graduate and beginning nursing students. College made R.N.s aware of nursing's second class status, contributed to their dissatisfaction, and gave them the tools to challenge their oppressors. Chapter 3 deals with the growth of collegiate nursing education and its impact on the women involved.

Endnotes

1. Louise Alcott, "Combining Marriage and Nursing," *AJN* 55 (November 1955): 1344.

2. Elinor Quandt, "Letters - Pro And Con," *AJN* 55 (October 1955): 1160.

3. Goldin, *Understanding the Gender Gap*, 17; Hartmann, "Women's Employment and the Domestic Ideal," 86; McLaughlin et al., *Changing Lives*, 94.

4. Cherlin, *Marriage, Divorce, Remarriage*, 50-51.

5. McLaughlin et al., *Changing Lives*, 96.

6. McLaughlin et al., *Changing Lives*, 56.

7. May, *Homeward Bound*, 6.

8. McLaughlin et al., *Changing Lives*, 127.

9. Cherlin, *Marriage, Divorce, Remarriage*, 22; May, *Homeward Bound*, 8.

10. Crispell, "Myths of the 1950s," 41; McLaughlin et al., *Changing Lives*, 126.

11. May, *Homeward Bound*, 155.

12. McLaughlin et al., *Changing Lives*, 126-131.

13. Cherlin, *Marriage, Divorce, Remarriage*, 20.

14. McLaughlin et al., *Changing Lives*, 60-61.

15. Klein, *Gender Politics*, 54-55, 60-61, 69-78.

16. Cherlin, *Marriage, Divorce, Remarriage*, 51; McLaughlin et al., *Changing Lives*, 50.

17. Cherlin, *Marriage, Divorce, Remarriage*, 50; Goldin, *Understanding the Gender Gap*, 174-176, 180-181.

18. Hartmann, "Women's Employment and the Domestic Ideal," 92-93.

19. Goldin, *Understanding the Gender Gap*, 176.

20. Jackson, *Crabgrass Frontier*, 4, 243; May, *Homeward Bound*, 77, 164-172.

21. Hartmann, "Women's Employment and the Domestic Idea," 86.

22. ANA, *Facts About Nursing 1950* (New York: ANA, 1950), 14; ANA, *Facts, 1968*, 16; Suzanne H. Friedman, "The Aging Nurse," *Nursing Outlook* 12 (November 1964): 25; Evelyn B. Moses, "The Profile of a Professional Nurse," *AJN* 60 (March 1960): 369; Margaret Ranck, "Our Readers Say," *Nursing Outlook* 1 (February 1953): 68.

23. Edna E. Sharritt, "Where are the ex-service nurses?" *AJN* 46 (December 1946): 850.

24. "5,000 Civilian Nurses," *AJN*, 45 (December 1945): 1020.

25. ANA, "Age, Marital Status, and Employment of Professional Registered Nurses," *AJN* 50 (February 1950): 68.

26. Burgess, *Nurses, Patients, and Pocketbooks*, 20, 37, 80; Melosh, *"The Physician' Hand,"* 41, 87; Reverby, *Ordered to Care*, 166, 170, 177-179.

27. Colonel Florence A. Blanchfield, AUS, Superintendent, ANC, "Letters - Pro And Con," *AJN* 46 (February 1946): 134; "News About Nursing," *AJN* 44 (December 1944): 1178; "Nursing - on V-E Day and Beyond," *AJN* 45 (June 1945): 424; "Urgent Need for Nurses," *AJN* 44 (November 1944): 1017; "With Army and Navy Nurses," *AJN* 46 (April 1946): 261-262.

28. ANA, *Facts About Nursing, 1955-56* (New York: ANA, 1956), 190; ANA, *Facts, 1964*, 244, 247; ANA, *Facts, 1968*, 222, 224, 227; Crispell, "Myths of the 1950s," 40.

29. Paul Starr, *The Social Transformation of American Medicine* (New York: Basic Books, Inc., 1982), 311-328; Rosemary Stevens, *In Sickness and Wealth: American Hospitals in the Twentieth Century* (New York: Basic Books, Inc., 1989), 231, 258, 281.

30. Starr, *Social Transformation of Medicine*, 335-336.

31. Starr, *Social Transformation of Medicine*, 335-344; Stevens, *In Sickness and Wealth*, 228.

32. Starr, *Social Transformation of Medicine*, 338, 348-350, 361; Stevens, *In Sickness and Wealth*, 228.

33. Starr, *Social Transformation of Medicine*, 335-364; Stevens, *In Sickness and Wealth*, 228-231.

34. Katherine J. Densford, "Address of the President," *American Nurses' Association Proceedings, Volume 1 - House of Delegates, Thirty-fifty Biennial Convention, September 22-27, 1946, Atlantic City, New Jersey*, 11.

35. Mary N. Roberts, "Nursing in 1947 and Beyond," *AJN* 48 (January 1948): 1.

36. Mary N. Roberts, "The Rich Report and the Crisis in Nursing," *AJN* 47 (April 1947): 208.

37. E.L. Bortz, "The Crisis in Nursing," *AJN* 47 (August 1947): 527.

38. "Continuing Shortage of Nurse Supply," *Nursing Outlook* 14 (July 1966): 8; "How Many Nurses," *AJN* 65 (February 1965): 24; "Increasing Numbers Fail to Alleviate Nurse Shortage," *AJN*, 66 (July 1966): 1464.

39. ANA, *Facts, 1959*, 16; ANA, *Facts, 1968*, 193; "News from Here And There," *Nursing Outlook* 15 (February 1967): 72.

40. Zella Bryant and Helen H. Hudson, "The Census of Nurses in Public Health," *AJN* 62 (December 1962): 104; Vera Freeman, "Staff Nurse Vacancies in Selected Public Health Nursing Agencies - 1961," *Nursing Outlook* 10 (February 1962): 112; Mildred Gaynor, "Public Health Nursing for the Future," *Nursing Outlook* 5 (July 1957): 399; "News Highlights," *AJN* 58 (April 1958): 494.

41. Lucile Petry Leone, "Where Will We Find Teachers?" *AJN* 55 (December 1955): 1461.

42. Martha Z. Belote, "Nurses and the Army Build-up," *AJN* 62 (February 1962): 84-85; "News," *AJN*, 64 (September 1964): 44.

43. "Four-Point Plan Proposed in New York," *AJN* 55 (June 1955): 732; Roberts, "The Rich Report," 208; "To Meet Our Nursing Needs," *AJN* 58 (September 1958): 1266.

44. Lily Mary David, "The Economic Status of the Nursing Profession," *AJN* 47 (July 1947): 456.

45. ANA, *Facts, 1961*, 80; "Professional Nursing School Admissions Decline in 1956," *AJN* 57 (August 1957): 1006.

46. ANA, "Calling American Nurses to Action," *Convention Journal* (April 26, 1954); Leone, "People, Nurses, and Students," 933; "Nurses for a Growing Nation," *AJN* 57 (June 1957): 771.

47. ANA, "Nurse Supply Vital Issue," *Convention Journal* (June 12, 1958); ANA, "Secretary Ribicoff Lauds Nurses, Cites Education Needs," *Convention Journal* (May 16, 1962): 1; Nell V. Beeby, "It's June Again," *AJN* 53 (June 1953): 673; Friedman, "The Aging Nurse," 25; NLN, "Must Plan Today To Solve Staffing Needs Tomorrow," *Convention Outlook* (April 13, 1961): 2; Mary Roberts, "Married Nurses," *AJN* 49 (November 1949): 680; Ranck, "Our Readers Say,"68.

48. David, "Economic Status," 458; Alice K. Leopold and Ewan Clague, "The BLS Survey," *AJN* 58 (September 1958): 1261; Mary M. Richardson, "This Pay Cafeteria Works," *AJN* 48 (August 1948): 496-497.

49. ANA, *Facts, 1952*, 18; ANA, *Facts About Nursing, 1960* (New York: ANA, 1960), 8; ANA, *Facts, 1968*, 20; ANA, *Facts, '74-'75*, 18.

50. Roberts, "Married Nurses," 680.

51. Ranck, "Our Readers Say," 68.

52. Friedman, "The Aging Nurse," 25.

53. Vernice Ferguson, "Come Back to Work!" *Nursing Outlook* 18 (October 1970): 58-59.

54. C.B., "Letters - Pro And Con," *AJN* 47 (April 1947): 255.

55. Ruth Roswal, "Letters - Pro And Con," *AJN* 52 (July 1952): 792.

56. Betty L. Houseman, "Letters to the Editor," *The Pennsylvania Nurse* 8 (March 1953): 3.

57. Reverby, *Ordered to Care*, 203-204.

58. Hannah Burggren, "Part-time Nurses Can Be an Asset," *AJN* 49 (November 1949): 681.

59. "Married Nurses and Hospital Staffing," *AJN* 53 (April 1953): 438-439.

60. Jane Wood, "Letters," *AJN* 66 (October 1966): 2176.

61. Helen L. McCarty, "Letters," *AJN* 64 (March 1964): 66.

62. Annabelle Peterson, "Report from the Committee on Nursing in National Defense," *AJN* 57 (May 1957): 605.

63. Grace M. McFadden, "The Part-Time Nurse in the School," *Nursing Outlook* 12 (October 1964): 62.

64. Mary Ann Staab, "Reclaim Those Lost Nurses!" *Nursing Outlook* 12 (October 1964): 605.

65. Jeanne R. Shaw, "Letters," *AJN* 70 (March 1970): 490.

66. ANA, *Facts, 1961*, 7; ANA, *Facts About Nursing, 1965* (New York: ANA, 1965), 7; Arthur Testoff, Eugene Levine, Stanley E. Siegal, "The Part-Time Nurse," *AJN* 64 (January 1964): 88-89.

67. ANA, *Facts About Nursing, 1969* (New York: ANA, 1969), 7.

68. ANA, *Facts About Nursing, 1954* (New York: ANA, 1954), 110; ANA, *Facts About Nursing, 1957* (New York: ANA, 1957), 116.

69. Marian Martin Pettengill, "Multilateral Collective Bargaining and the Health Care Industry: Implications for Nursing," *Journal of Professional Nursing* 1 (September-October 1985): 277.

70. ANA, *Facts, 1960*, 120, 132, 144, 151.

71. Evelyn Moses, "How Much Nurses Are Paid," *AJN* 61 (May 1961): 92.

72. ANA, *Facts, 1962-1963*, 133, 146, 152.

73. ANA, *Facts About Nursing, 1967* (New York: ANA, 1967), 137, 148, 154, 162; George Stelluto, "Earnings of Hospital Nurses, July 1966," *Monthly Labor Review* 90 (June 1967): 55-58.

74. Pettingill, "Multilateral Collective Bargaining," 276-277; "Salaries Up, Especially for General Duty," *AJN* 70 (June 1970): 1206.

75. ANA, *Facts About Nursing, 1970-71* (New York: ANA, 1971), 127-128, 142, 160.

76. ANA, *Facts, 1968*, 131, 143; ANA, *Facts, 1969*, 131, 138; ANA, *Facts, '72-'73*, 130-131, 136, 144, 156.

77. ANA, "Private Duty Opening Business Session," *American Nurses' Association Proceedings, Volume 1 - Advisory Council - Section Meetings - Joint And Special Sessions, Thirty-fifty Biennial Convention, September 22-27* (Atlantic City, New Jersey, 1946), 302, 331; ANA, "Executive Director's Report," *House Of Delegates Reports, 1966-1968, 46th Convention, American Nurses' Association* (Dallas, Texas, 1968), 26; "Urge Refreshers For 30,000 This Year," *AJN* 67 (March 1967): 471.

78. Jane Chips, "Letters," *AJN* 68 (February 1968): 263; Marion Pearce, "Something Really Refreshing," *AJN* 62 (February 1962): 98-99; Madeline Tabler, "Welcome Back To Nursing," *Nursing Outlook* 13 (September 1966): 67-68; Elizabeth Worley, "Monsters, Monitors, and the Merry Mouseketeers," *AJN* 69 (July 1969): 1443-1445.

79. Dorothy E. Reese, D. Ann Sparmacher, Arthur Testoff, "How Many Caps Went On Again?" *Nursing Outlook* 10 (August 1962): 517.

80. Helen C. Anderson, "Refreshed Will Work Part-Time," *AJN* 68 (October 1968): 2188-2189.

81. Anderson, "Refreshed Will Work," 2189; Pearce, "Something Really Refreshing," 98; Reese, Sparmacher, Testoff, "How Many Caps," 519.

82. Tabler, "Welcome Back To Nursing," 68.

83. Joy DeLeon, "Letters - Pro And Con," *AJN* 55 (July 1955): 776.

84. Reese, Sparmacher, and Testoff, "How Many Caps," 519.

85. Dorothy E. Reese, Stanley E. Siegel, Arthur Testoff, "The Inactive Nurse," *AJN* 64 (November 1964): 125.

86. ANA, *Facts, 1954*, 91; "If You Ask Me," *AJN* 59 (June 1959): 810-811.

87. Helen F. Callon and Margaret Farrell, "The Pregnant Hospital Employee," *AJN* 63 (May 1963): 111.

88. "If You Ask Me," 810-811.

89. Lois Bookman, "Letters - Pro And Con," *AJN* 50 (August 1950): 4.

90. George C. Schicks, "Hospital Turns Baby Sitter," *Nursing Outlook* 2 (November 1954): 574-575.

91. "Day Care Services Help Recruit Nurses," *AJN* 63 (September 1963): 97-100.

92. Luella Samuelson, "Our Summer Day Nursery," *AJN* 52 (July 1952): 871.

93. Pauline Stack Cooper, "A Successful Venture in Day Nursery Care," *AJN* 59 (March 1959): 365.

94. "Hospital Day Care Centers Pay Off, Survey Finds," *AJN* 70 (December 1970): 2630, 2632.

95. Everett C. Hughes, Helen MacGill Hughes, and Irwin Deutscher, *Twenty Thousand Nurses Tell Their Story* (Philadelphia: J.B. Lippincott Company, 1958), 185.

96. Barbara G. Schutt, "The Birds in the Hand," *AJN* 63 (April 1963): 57.

97. Anderson, "Refreshed Will Work," 2189.

98. For a discussion of the training school as an agent of socialization see Melosh, *"The Physician's Hand,"* 47-67; Tomes, " 'Little World of Our Own,' " 478.

99. Melosh, *"The Physician's Hand,"* 66.

100. Hughes, Hughes, and Deutscher, *Twenty Thousand Nurses*, 49-60.

101. Susan Gortner, "Nursing Majors in Twelve Western Universities: A Comparison Of Registered Nurse Students And Basic Senior Students," *Nursing Research* 17 (March-April 1968): 127.

102. "Did We Say 'Inactive?' " *Nursing Outlook* 10 (November 1962): 721.

103. "They Donned Their Caps Again,"*AJN* 52 (July 1952): 842.

104. "They Donned Their Caps Again," 842.

105. S.M., "Letters - Pro And Con," *AJN* 47 (April 1974): 255.

106. Marian D. Austin, "Letters - Pro And Con," *AJN* 53 (December 1953): 1414.

107. "Inactive Nurse Sets Up Pre-Refresher Course," *AJN* 67 (February 1967): 254.

108. Elyse M. Rogers, "Letters," *AJN* 65 (February 1965): 59.

109. Mary Lou Baloun, "Letters," *AJN* 64 (November 1964): 58.

110. Jane Woods, "Letters," *AJN* 66 (October 1966): 2176.

111. Joanne W. Urstadt, "Letters," *AJN* 69 (August 1969): 1638.

112. Mary C. Fischelis and Nancy H. French, "Three Full-Time Jobs: Nurse, Wife, and Mother," *AJN* 68 (January 1968): 76, 78.

113. Jean Gaylord, "Letters," *AJN* 68 (October 1968): 2118.

114. Chips, "Letters," 263.

115. Worley, "Monsters," 1444.

116. Anderson, "Refreshed Will Work," 2189; Lucille Knopf, *Registered Nurses Fifteen Years After Graduation* (New York: NLN, 1983), 21; Moses, "Profile," 369; Christopher A. Webb, "The Nurse Today - '68," *RN* 31 (July 1968): 43.

117. ANA, *Facts, 1968,* 20, 22.

118. Lucie Young Kelly, "The New Breed," *Nursing Outlook* 29 (July 1981): 440.

CHAPTER 3:

Refueling the Lamp:
Nursing and College Education, 1950-1985

In 1966 Alma Woolley earned a master's degree from the University of Pennsylvania School of Nursing. One year later the *AJN* published her account of graduate school. Woolley spoke glowingly of her experience. College had afforded her in-depth knowledge of nursing, the opportunity to learn educational theory and practice, and the self-confidence gained from completing a demanding course of study. In her enthusiasm Woolley used a symbol well-known to nurses — Florence Nightingale's famous lantern. "My lamp," Woolley wrote, "is refueled."[1]

College attendance was an increasingly common aspect of women's lives after World War II. In 1940 only ten percent of women aged 24 to 29 had completed at least one year of college. By 1960 it had risen to fifteen percent. The proportion soared to forty percent by 1980. Between 1964 and 1984 the percentage of female college graduates in this age group doubled. Gaps between men and women also narrowed. The ratio of female to male college graduates was .56 in 1960. It rose to .71 in 1970 and .85 in 1981.[2] Economic prosperity, expansion of the service sector, the end of the marriage bar, public financial support, and affirmative action all fueled this growth.[3] Higher education opened up new worlds, particularly for baby boomers. Graduates from this generation embarked on careers and delayed marriage and child-rearing more often than any earlier group of American women.[4] Dissatisfied, college-educated females played major roles in the re-emergence of the women's movement.[5]

Entering college was also a common theme in nursing between 1950 and the mid-1980s. Both hospital-trained R.N.s and women fresh out of high school enrolled in community colleges and universities. Hospital schools first experienced declining enrollments during the

1950s. After 1970 they educated less than a quarter of American nursing students (See Figure 6). Numerous professional, political, and social trends encouraged this educational migration. By the 1970s the percentage of nurses with college degrees had risen markedly, paralleling wider societal trends in female educational attainment. Like other American women, nurses also found that college attendance changed them. College-educated R.N.s viewed themselves, the health care system, and their society differently.

**FIGURE 6: PERCENTAGE OF NURSING STUDENTS
ENROLLED IN VARIOUS ENTRY-LEVEL
EDUCATIONAL PROGRAMS, 1940-1980[a]**

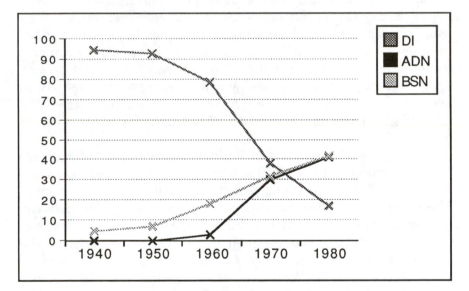

Note: Students enrolled in DI (Diploma) programs attended two or three
          year hospital schools. ADN (Associate Degree in Nursing) students
          attended two year community colleges. Those studying for a BSN
          (Bachelor of Science Degree in Nursing) were enrolled in four year
          college or university programs.

   a.   *Sources:* ANA, *Facts, 1951*, 41; ANA, *Facts About Nursing, '76-'77*
        (Kansas City: ANA, 1977), 97; ANA, *Facts About Nursing, '80-'81*
        (New York: AJN Company, 1981), 152.

Changes in health care delivery loomed large among the factors encouraging nurses' college attendance. Postwar medical technology transformed nursing practice. R.N.s who administered new drug thera-pies, cared for complicated surgical cases, and worked in intensive care units and emergency rooms had to be scientifically literate. As Esther Lucille Brown, author of a 1947 report pointed out, hospital staff nurses made complex, split-second decisions concerning patients' treatments. They needed, therefore, to be educated as physicians' colleagues rather than handmaidens.[6] Jobs outside the hospital also required new pro-fessional skills. As a Pennsylvania director of nursing observed, R.N.s in public health, administration, and education needed a good back-ground in human relations, evaluation techniques, teaching skills, prin-ciples of supervision, community responsibility and participation, methods of research or approaches to the use of research findings.[7]

The evolution of emergency care for cardiac patients illustrates the way in which medical advances changed nursing. In the early 1960s closed-chest heart massage became a viable treatment. Health care pro-fessionals debated who should learn and use the new technique. The American Heart Association recommended that only M.D.s initiate the procedure. But physicians increasingly delegated to nurses and R.N.s spent more time close to patients. Nurses recognized they would ulti-mately be the ones to administer closed-chest massage. As *AJN* editor Barbara Schutt wrote in a 1961 editorial, "Reality reminds us that, even in a hospital, it is rare to have a physician available to a patient within three minutes."[8] Hospitals arrived at the same conclusions and taught closed-chest massage to registered nurses.

This situation presented nurses with new responsibilities. It enabled them to perform a technique originally designated for doctors. It also required them to make decisions independently and quickly. Often as not R.N.s, not M.D.s, determined whether cardiac arrest had occurred and started treatment.[9] Later in the decade cardiac resuscitation, and nurses' role in the process, became even more sophisticated. R.N.s monitored, defibrilated, and used other complex lifesaving measures. As had been true earlier with closed-chest massage, nurses worked autonomously. In the words of Barbara Melosh,

> No critical care nurse would call a doctor to report meekly, "Mr Brown's pulse appears to have ceased." She would yell for emergency equipment, pound the patient's chest, inflate his lungs, initiate closed-chest cardiac mas-sage, perhaps even begin to administer the drugs used in resuscitation.[10]

Increasingly postwar America required new types of nurses. The hospital schools were not able, however, to provide them. Apprentice-ship training, particularly in small general hospitals, did not prepare

R.N.s for the demands of modern practice. Nurses were now more than care-givers. They were also health teachers, problem solvers, and even healers. To fulfill these roles they had to study areas the hospital schools neglected — the liberal arts, the social sciences, decision-making, and critical thinking. These areas composed the curriculum of the modern university. In order to perform competently, postwar nurses needed college degrees.

By the late 1940s professional associations began to call for sweeping changes in nurses' training. As mentioned in Chapter 1, earlier attempts at educational reform had focused on closing smaller and inferior hospital schools. Now nursing leaders advocated moving programs into institutions of higher education. They maintained that only colleges and universities could properly teach women about sophisticated health care delivery and nurses' multi-faceted roles.[11] They also argued that educating R.N.s in colleges helped solve the shortage, particularly in public health, education and administration. Employers in these areas preferred candidates with graduate degrees. Nurses with hospital diplomas had to complete two college programs before they could fill these critical jobs.[12] As early as 1951 NLN president, Agnes Gelinas, reasoned that educating beginning students in four-year colleges shortened the time necessary to produce nurse-specialists.[13] In 1957 the NLN likewise stated that entry-level college education was the most efficient way to train teachers, administrators, supervisiors, and clinical specialists.[14]

Nursing leaders saw college education as a means of securing the status and autonomy they had craved since the 1880s. The ANA leadership, much influenced by the work of sociologist Robert K. Merton, argued that apprenticeship education was a barrier to professional recognition. Society granted status and autonomy to certain occupations based on their level of expertise. In twentieth century America "expertise" came in large part from possession of a college degree.[15] Loretta Heidgerken, a Catholic University nursing professor, writing in 1969, agreed with this assessment.

> Almost without a dissenting voice, those who know the trends in professional education in the United States agree that the preparation of the professional person belongs in the college or university. It follows, then, that the preparation of the professional nurse also belongs there.[16]

Furthermore, as an educational consultant noted, nurses could not "meet on equal terms with persons in other professions" unless they, too, held college degrees.[17]

The nursing associations were well aware that college had become more accessible for middle and working class Americans. The leadership therefore feared they would lose potential students if hospital schools continued to educate R.N.s. As early as 1949 Agnes Gelinas observed that "nursing would be wise to structure a developmental and integrated four-year college program."[18] That same year Mary Roberts reminded *AJN* readers that "nursing must compete for students, with an increasingly wide variety of professions and occupations."[19] In the 1950s, NLN statistics showed a decrease in the proportion of female high school graduates entering nursing. The professional press blamed this on the lack of collegiate programs.[20] Nursing leaders feared that the quality, as well as quantity, would suffer from the continuation of apprenticeship training. Rutgers University's Hildegard Peplau issued this warning in 1966. "In another decade, if nursing remains the only 'profession' trained in noneducational service institutions, it will not recruit from the top forty percent of high school graduates."[21] Margaret Brown Harty, the NLN's Director of the Division of Nursing Education, echoed Peplau's concerns in 1968.

> The young woman high school graduate seeking to achieve a helping role may be attracted to nursing. Conversely, she may be repulsed by the prospect of traditional rituals, regimenting uniforms, or confining schedules [of the hospital schools].[22]

Americans found college more accessible, in large part, because increased public spending made higher education affordable. Framed as a means of gradually easing veterans back into the work force, the Servicemen's Adjustment Acts of 1944 and 1952 provided tuition and monthly subsistence for G.I.s who wanted to attend college.[23] After the Soviet Union launched its Sputnik satellite in 1957, Americans feared an "education gap" and demanded that the government take action. The subsequent National Defense Education Act of 1958 provided $1 billion in loans and scholarships for college students majoring in math, science, engineering, and foreign languages. During the 1960s Congress granted additional funds for higher education as part of Lyndon Johnson's Great Society program.[24]

Nursing organizations, aware of this trend, lobbied the federal government on behalf of their own educational programs. Because of the chronic R.N. shortage, professional associations could make a good case for public support. The first government programs for nursing education benefitted graduate students. In 1948 the National Institute of Mental Health, concerned about the psychological problems of veterans, awarded research grants and traineeships to colleges which prepared psychiatric nurses. The Health Amendments Act of 1956 established endowments for masters and doctoral students in nursing education and administration. By 1961 graduate nursing students could apply for public health and Children's Bureau traineeships. Low interest loans were also available from the National Defense Student Loan Program. During these same years twelve states released funds for graduate nursing education.[25]

By the mid-1960s the associations also lobbied successfully for aid to undergraduate programs. In 1964 Congress passed the landmark Nurse Training Act. The NTA authorized funds for nursing school construction, scholarships, and loans. Along with renewing the NTA five times, Congress passed additional legislation. Nursing received scholarship funds under both the 1966 Nursing Education Opportunity Grant Act and the 1968 Health Manpower Act.[26] State governments, responding the nursing shortage, also passed scholarship aid packages in the 1960s.[27]

Federal and state aid enabled colleges to both build and expand nursing education programs. Between 1965 and 1985 the number of schools offering the BSN more than doubled. Associate degree programs increased eightfold (See Figure 7). Thousands of American nursing students benefitted from government-financed scholarships, grants, and loans. Seventy-seven percent of the undergraduates who received NTA money during the 1960s came from families with annual incomes of less than $10,000. Similarly, forty percent of NIMH grant recipients could not have attended graduate school without aid. [28]

Besides lobbying for public funding, the professional associations investigated the feasibility of developing community college programs. First established as private, sectarian institutions in the nineteenth century, two year colleges had become increasingly popular in the early twentieth.[29] Community colleges, many publicly funded, offered classes for students not ready for the university, along with terminal, vocational coursework. They provided job training for the unemployed in the 1930s and war-related, technical instruction during World War II. In 1941 200,000 students attended 560 community colleges, primarily in Midwestern and Western states.[30]

After World War II community colleges, like four-year institutions, grew phenomenally. Two-year schools expanded to service veterans interested in occupational training. Public policy favored community colleges as well. In 1948 both the President's Commission on Higher

FIGURE 7: U.S. NURSING SCHOOLS, 1945-1985[a]

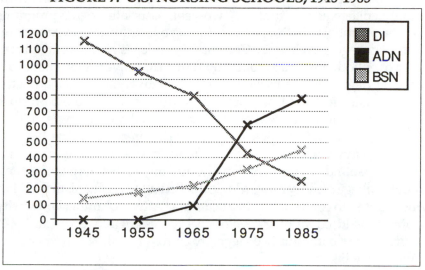

Note: The number of ADN programs for 1955 is included with those for BSN schools.

a.   *Sources:* ANA, *Facts About Nursing, 1945* (New York: ANA, 1945), 30-31; ANA, *Facts, 1955-56,* 90; ANA, *Facts About Nursing, 1966* (New York: ANA, 1966), 93; ANA, *Facts About Nursing, 86-87* (New York: ANA, 1987), 32; Walter L. Johnson, "Educational Preparation for Nursing - 1975," *Nursing Outlook* 24 (September 1976): 569.

Education for Democracy and California's Strayer Report urged states to expand two-year, post-secondary schools. Publicly funded community colleges, they believed, had the potential to make higher education universally available and fiscally efficient. Proponents saw community colleges as institutions which could provide general education, terminal degree programs, and support for students who would eventually transfer to a four-year school. Community colleges were attractive to adult students as well new high school graduates. In the 1960s, 1970s, and 1980s these schools recruited minority and disabled students, as well as their former constituencies.[31] As states passed enabling legislation and governments at all levels allocated funds, the numbers of facilities and students mushroomed. In 1948 500,00 students attended 580 community colleges. The figures for 1968 were 2 million and 993, respectively.[32] In 1985 the United States contained 1,000 community colleges which enrolled one-third of all post-secondary students.[33]

Nursing educators wasted no time in allying themselves with community college administrators. Two-year, associate degree programs had the potential to both upgrade nursing education and expand community college enrollments. Community colleges had several advantages over both hospital schools and four-year universities. First of all, associate degree programs were low cost, relatively short, and attracted older female students from local communities. They could produce nurses, many of whom could not have attended another type of institution, quickly and inexpensively. Secondly, freed from the hospital school's heavy workloads, ADN students learned nursing in an educationally sound enviroment. Finally, nursing leaders hoped the community college could serve as a logical articulation mechanism for R.N.s who wanted to continue their education.[34] After Columbia University professor Mildred Montag developed a successful pilot project in 1952, the number of community college programs and ADN students grew rapidly (See Figures 6 and 7).[35]

As programs developed and funds became available, college proponents argued that the climate for educational reform had never been better. During the 1960s the professional associations took strong and definitive stances on the issue. The ANA's Committee on Current and Long-Term Goals proposed, in 1960, that all professional nurses be educated in baccalaureate programs.[36] In May 1965 NLN convention delegates passed Resolution 5. This policy "recognized and strongly supported the trend toward collegiate nursing."[37] That same year the ANA Board of Directors issued "The 1965 Position Paper on Education." It endorsed the following proposals.

> The education for all those who are licensed to practice nursing should take place in institutions of higher education. Minimum preparation for beginning professional nursing practice at the present time should be baccalaureate degree eduction in nursing. Minimum preparation for beginning technical [bedside] nursing practice at the present time should be associate degree education in nursing.[38]

Many hospital school graduates, fearful that educational reform downgraded their own credentials, tried to overturn the NLN/ANA positions.[39] Other women saw the new trends as opportunities. The professional associations' endorsements encouraged licensed nurses to attend college. Fifty-three percent of the R.N.s enrolled in one New England university, for example, returned to school in response to the Position Paper and Resolution 5.[40] Similarly two Pittsburgh hospital graduates enrolled in local colleges during 1966 and 1968, convinced apprenticeship training handicapped their careers.[41] In an attempt to encourage nurses, BSN schools relaxed admission and credit transfer requirements, promoted "open curriculum" programs, and scheduled classes for the convenience of employed students.[42] Increasingly large numbers of colleges and universities accepted R.N.s with hospital diplomas (See Figure 8).

FIGURE 8: NURSING EDUCATION PROGRAMS ACCEPTING R.N.S, 1956-1980[a]

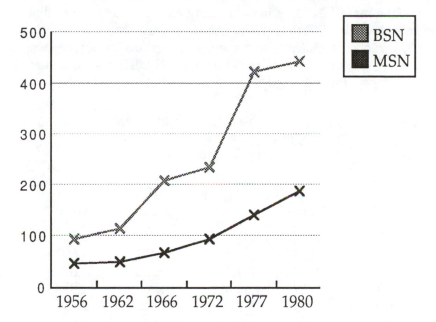

Note: MSN refers to Master of Science in Nursing.

   a.   Sources: ANA, *Facts About Nursing, 1958* (New York: ANA, 1958), 96; ANA, *Facts, 1964,* 116, 122; ANA, *Facts, 1967,* 126, 128; ANA, *Facts, '74-'75,* 91, 93; ANA, *Facts , '80-'81,* 164, 166; ANA, *Facts About Nursing, '82-'83* (New York: ANA, 1983), 72, 175.

Official endorsements about college education also influenced the choices of entry-level students. One public health nurse recalled visiting a New Jersey hospital school with her parents in 1966. There, an instructor informed them about the Position Paper and advised her to attend college.[43] Another young woman, approaching high school graduation in 1974, became aware of the new educational trends through her mother who was an R.N. She enrolled in the University of Pennsylvania's School of Nursing because she believed the BSN made her more marketable.[44]

Because of the trends discussed above, the number of women enrolled in collegiate nursing schools greatly expanded. Less than seven percent of entry-level students attended college in 1950. By 1980 slightly over eighty percent of nursing students enrolled in ADN and BSN programs (Se Figure 6). The number of hospital graduates who earned college degrees also increased rapidly after 1970 (See Figure 9). At mid-decade the rate of increase in continuing education exceeded that of the entry-level. In 1978 the NLN stated that "basic [entry-level] education has reached a plateau," but masters programs showed a twelve percent growth rate.[45] In the mid-1980s, while basic enrollments fell, post-entry programs thrived.[46]

FIGURE 9: REGISTERED NURSE ENROLLMENTS AND GRADUATIONS FROM BSN AND MSN PROGRAMS, 1955-1985[a]

	BSN Enroll.	BSN Grad.	MSN Enroll.	MSN Grad.
1955	9,572	1,935	1,757	528
1960	9,609	2,520	1,424	1,092
1965	9,021	2,254	3,123	1,379
1970	7,692	2,413	4,443	1,988
1975	15,854	3,791	9,662	2,694
1980	28,033	7,365	15,053	4,778
1985	41,808	9,794	18,973	5,321

a. *Sources:* ANA, *Facts, 1957,* 88; ANA, *Facts, 1961,* 110, 114; ANA, *Facts, 1964,* 117; ANA, *Facts, 1966 ,* 102, 104; ANA, *Facts, 1969,* 109; ANA, *Facts About Nursing, '70-'71* (New York: ANA, 1971), 106; ANA, *Facts, '72-'73,* 109; ANA, *Facts About Nursing, '76-'77* (Kansas City: ANA, 1977), 121; ANA, *Facts, '82-'83,* 168; ANA, *Facts, 86-87,* 53, 57; Johnson, "Educational Preparation - 1975," 570-571.

These changing educational trends had significant consequences for nursing. As college enrollments increased, the educational profiles of employed nurses changed dramatically. The 1951 Inventory of Registered Professional Nurses, the first to report on educational levels, found that only 8.2 percent of active nurses had a bachelors or masters degree.[47] In 1962 and 1972, 10.0 and 17.5 percent of employed R.N.s possessed a BSN or MSN. In the latter year 14.3 percent had earned an ADN.[48] By 1980 the proportion of nurses with an associate degree was 20.1. Another 23.1 and 5.1 percent had bachelors and masters degrees. In 1980 .8 percent possessed a Ph.D or Ed.D.[49]

Nursing's entry into higher education also had a significance which transcended numbers of students and degrees. Nurses who attended college developed new competencies, skills, and attitudes. Unquestionably they learned more about nursing. Continuing education students in particular benefitted from the university experience. One clinical specialist believed the opportunities she received in her masters program — participation in research, grant money, and collaboration with experts in her field — greatly enhanced her nursing practice.[50] In her 1967 article Alma Woolley testified about the effectiveness of her own graduate education.

> Certainly I accomplished my main objective, to learn about the process of nursing education itself. Courses in both the school of education and the school of nursing made me familiar with philosophies and methods and helped me to develop my own. Practice teaching gave me the confidence I sorely needed to face a class of college level students. As in many other areas, there is no substitute for experience, but there is also no substitute for careful examination of the facts and theory.[51]

A nursing instructor at the Medical College of Virginia, who like Woolley earned an MSN in the 1960s, agreed. "The courses," she stated, "enriched my teaching."[52] The college experience also helped R.N.s interested in general, bedside nursing. In the words of one who entered a BSN program after fifteen years of practice,

> I *am* [italics hers] one of the elite: I give better patient care, I see each patient-family unit in a truer perspective, and I feel the sense of well-being when I can give more because I have learned more. [53]

Entry-level students benefitted immensely from higher education. In community colleges and universities, students were freed from the service requirements of the hospital schools. While apprenticeship education had enabled nurses to practice manual skills, many knew little about nursing theory or related subjects. As one R.N. had argued in 1967, "In many instances [hospital school education] is not education at all. Instead student nurses are staffing the hospitals."[54] Many students had resented the long hours and heavy workloads of the training schools. As two northeastern Pennsylvania nurses explained, "It seemed like we [the students] did all the work because we did!"[55]

College students, however, learned more than nursing theory and practice. They exhibited a sense of professionalism quite different from that of hospital-trained R.N.s. Research studies found that associate and baccalaureate degree students scored significantly higher in autonomy and patient advocacy than those from hospital schools. College students also disagreed more openly with physicians and supervisors.[56]

College-educated nurses exhibited these attitudes because the climate at their schools was very different from that of the hospital. During interviews, training school graduates continually emphasized that, as students, they had no rights. One, for example, had suffered verbal abuse from physicians. During a particularly painful incident a surgeon unjustly reprimanded her, because she reminded him that he had left a needle in a patient.[57] A classmate experienced mistreatment from both M.D.s and R.N.s. On one occasion an obnoxious surgeon stuffed a towel down her scrub dress. Her pharmacology instructor yelled so much, nervous students found it impossible to pour medications without spilling them.[58] Another woman, a student at a nearby hospital, experienced sexual harassment at the hands of doctors. She had difficulty warding off these attacks because the school had trained her to be subservient.[59]

College students, on the other hand, were socialized to be autonomous practitioners rather than handmaidens. Fourteen hospital staff nurses, who wrote a 1962 article on doctor-nurse conflict, observed that college programs emphasized "independent functions."[60] Four years later Hildegard Peplau agreed with this assessment. "These [college-educated] nurses," she remarked, "have an image of the professional nurse as a competent independent practitioner...."[61]

College prepared R.N.s to behave as patient advocates. As one hospital staff nurse explained, the BSN curriculum made her more knowledgeable about patients' needs.

> When a patient questions the usefulness of a third I.V. that contains electrolytes, I can say more than "the doctor ordered it" or "it will make you feel better." The academics help me to know why a patient fights back when a Levin tube is inserted so I can solve the problem on that level.[62]

College socialized students to approach physicians differently. A Yale University MSN recalled that her professors continually stressed that nurses' primary responsiblity was to the patient. The Yale faculty encouraged students to question doctors and refuse incorrect orders.[63] By graduation college-educated R.N.s were firmly convinced of their ability to give patient-centered care. A director of nursing, in 1966, went so far as to insist that nurses were actually better able to meet clients' needs than M.D.s.[64]

As a result of their socialization, college-educated nurses saw themselves as physicians' colleagues. Faculty members specifically told their students not to practice hospital school rituals, such as standing when an M.D. entered the room.[65] College instructors did not allow medical staff to treat nursing students like "teenage idiots."[66] Nurses thus graduated from college with a strong sense of their own self-worth. As Hildegard Peplau noted,

> Nurses who hold graduate degrees tend to publish, to want to work directly with patients, to get out of the stereotype of the nurse as dowdy, compliant, but helpful to the doctor. These nurses have an image of the professional nurse as a competent, independent practitioner who discusses with the doctor, as a colleague, the need of patients and how these can best be met by interdisciplinary collaboration.[67]

Furthermore, as a nursing association official observed, college "made nurses more educationally equal" to university-trained physicians.[68]

The university also provided nurses with an avenue for learning "leadership skills in a nonthreatening environment."[69] Apprenticeship training rarely gave women this opportunity. Instead, hospital schools taught compliance and rigidly controlled behavior. Hospital students faced endless restrictions on their personal lives. One nurse, trained in a small mining community hospital, had particularly resented the strict curfew. Nursing students had to be indoors at an hour when school-age children played throughout the neighborhood.[70] Another disliked her school's dress code. The hospital required nursing students to wear girdles so that they wouldn't "jiggle" when they worked on the wards. The nursing director thumped the girls' buttocks every morning as a means of enforcing the rule.[71]

Community and four-year colleges had more liberal policies on student dress and conduct. They also helped students develop analytical, organizational, and interpersonal skills. College-educated nurses, particularly those at the upper levels, interacted with supportive and nurturing faculty, debated nursing issues, and participated in advanced level seminars.[72] As one remarked, "College graduates learned to think and question."[73] In a 1976 editorial *Nursing Outlook* editor, Edith Patton

Lewis, recalled how her Yale education enhanced her leadership skills and self-confidence.

> Our faculty took our maturity for granted, pitched their teaching accordingly, and accepted our variations in learning styles and approaches to care. We could question if we wanted to, object, criticize. We were listened to.[74]

Because of these experiences, college graduates became nursing's new leaders and activists. As a Mississipi BSN explained,

> I feel that my program of education very adequately prepared me to function given "the way it really is," to analyze current circumstances and work thorugh the system to be a change agent.[75]

During interviews nurses pointed to numerous instances where the skills they learned in college propelled them into leadership roles. One became a professional association officer almost immediately after being hired at a public health agency.[76] A clinical specialist was elected local association president at a large, university-affiliated medical center within a year of her employment. She served several terms and negotiated a number of contracts.[77] A third successfully fought understaffing in the county health department where she worked as an administrator.[78]

A large number of these students, particularly those who were older and already licensed, combined college with child-rearing. After lecturing a senior seminar in 1979, nursing leader Lucie Young Kelly was struck by the large number of mothers enrolled in the class.[79] Young's impressions were accurate. Nursing researchers found, particularly after 1975, that half of R.N. students were married and one-third were mothers. Their median ages ranged from thirty-two to forty.[80]

Wives and mothers who attended college learned to balance their studies and family demands in a way quite different from their peers who re-entered the nursing labor force. College level studies, even if undertaken on a part-time basis, required extensive out-of-class preparation. This took a larger degree of commitment than working a partial shift or serving as a weekend relief nurse. Women who managed households, while studying for exams and writing term papers, participated in a constant and stressful juggling act. As Alma Woolley explained,

> While my classmates could afford to spend an hour or two between classes in the lounge with coffee and cigarettes, commiserating about how much work they had to do, I sat in the library making headway on the bibliography. When they took an hour for a leisurely lunch or supper, I either ate a sandwich from a machine or did not eat at all, so that I cold do most of my reading in the time I had to spend in school. While they could get together

during the evening to plan and discuss assignments, I worked at home....
While my homemaker friends watched television, sewed, and baked cook-
ies for PTA, I narrowed my activities to the business at hand. From the minute
the children were tucked in, I read, wrote, and studied.[81]

While Woolley's husband supported her efforts, other women were
not so fortunate. One New York nursing professor, writing in 1979,
was impressed by the number of married students who persevered in
spite of spouses' objections.

The writer has listened to so many nursing students who are distressed,
referred a number of them to counselors, and has also seen a number of
marriages end in separation after about a year in the nursing program. There
are students who are beaten, care plans torn up and texts thrown the the
garbage by angry husbands who want more time and attention from their
wives. It is so painful to see a price paid because the woman wants more
education.[82]

Despite these difficulties wives and mothers found they could complete degrees without harming their families. Some maintained that
college attendance helped their children and enhanced family relationships. One mother proudly observed, six months before her graduation, "One byproduct [of her education] is the self-reliance and independence my sons, 12 and 8, are developing."[83] Kathryn Lewis made a
similar argument in a 1973 article.

My education itself is very much a family affair. I do believe Ed [her hus-
band] could challenge some of the courses he has helped me with. The children used tinker toy models to help me learn molecular structure. There has
been a great deal of sharing and mutual enthusiasm - a family commitment.[84]

Women who successfully combined college and family life emerged
from school with a belief that mothers could be professionally
commited. They did not qualify their professional activities in the same
way as the employed nurses discussed in Chapter 2. Alma Woolley's
response to a critical acquaintance illustrates the attitudes of nontraditional nursing students.

Very recently I was asked by someone who had apparently already decided
that I reject my womanly role, "Well I guess you would rather work than
stay home and be a wife and mother, wouldn't you?" I replied, as always,
"Not at all; I want to do both."[85]

College-educated nurses, particularly in the late 1960s and early
1970s, also witnessed political turmoil and student activism. Influenced
by the civil rights and nuclear disarmament movements, college students sought to transform American society. These young people were
sharply critical of both Cold War policy and conventional liberalism.

They argued that mass participation was necessary to fight poverty and injustice. College students joined groups such as the Student Non-violent Coordinating Committee (SNCC) and Students for a Democratic Society (SDS). They registered Southern black voters, organized urban welfare recipients, and protested the Vietnam War. Long hair and blue jeans became symbols of dissidence. Campus life erupted with student strikes and violence. A highly visible youth culture, associated with sex, drugs, and rock-and-roll music, burst on the American scene.[86]

At universities nurses came into contact with this student culture, broader and more diverse than that of the hospital schools. Nursing students interacted with faculty and classmates concerned with injustice and dedicated to changing the status quo. As they participated in campus life, these women became aware of social problems and involved in reform movements. A variety of experiences raised their consciousness. One graduate student credited some friends, majoring in history, with enlightening her about social issues.[87] An entry-level student was profoundly influenced by a philosophy professor active in the civil rights movement.[88] A third nurse recalled that participation in student government and late night dormitory debates heightened her awareness.[89] Formal educational experiences also politicized nursing students. As a Rutgers professor commented after teaching a public health course,

> They [nursing students] come in contact with human suffering, poverty, ignorance, and neglect, often to an extent which taxes their endurance. While the issues associated with these conditions may be somewhat theoretical to some liberal arts students, they are painfully real to nursing students...[90]

Many young women saw social activism as a natural extension of nursing. As one student wrote in a 1969 article, expertise in areas such as public health gave R.N.s the knowledge and skills necessary to fight injustice.[91] A Southern student urged, one year later, that nurses not "hide behind their white uniforms."[92] Another argued that the student movement's principles, "peace on earth, brotherhood, and objection to the hostility to one's fellows," were fully compatible with nursing ethics. She insisted that nurses could not become "well-rounded professional practitioners"until they "incorporated them [above-mentioned principles] into their lives and practices."[93]

As one might expect, much of nursing students' activism dealt with medical care and related issues. Students saw themselves as health advocates for the poor. They tried to use their expertise to both help the disadvantaged and affect public policy.[94] Nursing students from Texas

Woman's University, for example, spearheaded a 1968 movement to establish a free clinic in Houston's worst slum.[95] Three years later students testified about health care delivery at a U.S. Senate Labor and Public Welfare Committee hearing.[96] Through the National Student Nurses' Association college-going women performed volunteer work in Appalachia, participated in rallies and demonstrations, and lobbied for family planning and environmental legislation.[97]

As nursing students participated in campus life, they also began to exhibit uncharacteristic militance. Edith Patton Lewis surmised in 1969 that this was a natural consequence of the move into the university. "Nursing students," she reminded her readers, "are part of the academic community and are embroiled in its affairs."[98] Like students in other disciplines, nurses protested and participated in civil disobedience. San Francisco State College and Rutgers University nursing students boycotted classes during campus-wide strikes in 1968.[99] In 1970 those at Arizonia State University organized enviromental teach-ins.[100] After the slaying of four Kent State students that same year, BSNs at the University of Maryland demonstrated. Nursing majors at Howard University attended anti-war rallies.[101]

Young nurses also incorporated the rhetoric and tactics of the student movement into demands for educational reform. Nursing students wanted rights for themselves as well as justice for the poor. They argued that people enrolled in higher education had a right to help determine university policy. Liberal and radical students were upset with what they believed was undue timidity and conservatism in nursing education departments and associations. They, therefore, asserted their right to affect professional change.

By the end of the 1960s the nursing press reported several instances of student militance over educational policy. The Student Nurses' Association of Florida, for example, roundly criticized the state's community college presidents for their 1969 decision not to seek NLN accreditation. The students believed such action jeopardized funding and quality education.[102] Los Angeles City College nursing majors, faced with a similar situation, overrode administrative objections and sought national accreditation on their own.[103] In 1971 and 1972 the National Student Nurses' Association displayed uncharacteristic militance. It asked for clarification of "The Position Paper on Education" and issued statements declaring its independence from the ANA and NLN.[104] The most widely publicized incident of student rebellion occurred at Rutgers University's College of Nursing in 1968. For one week students boycotted clinical assignments to protest university funding policies. They also demanded representation on nursing faculty committees.[105] Irate instructors, who interpreted this behavior as irresponsible, confronted the boycott's leaders. The young women responded,

> by working to assure optimal educational preparation for ourselves and future nursing students at Rutgers we would not be disavowing our professional responsibility, but would be exercising it to the fullest.[106]

As nurses protested, studied, and otherwise participated in college life, their experiences had important implications for the profession. Education in academic settings encouraged a commitment to nursing as a career. One can argue that licensed R.N.s entered college with some sense of professional commitment. But the university experience — acquisition of a wider knowledge base, growth of self-confidence, development of leaderships skills, and the realization that one could balance work and family — certainly promoted and reinforced career orientation.

Furthermore, colleges socialized entry-level students differently than the hospital schools.Like their colleagues in continuing education programs, ADN and BSN students had the opportunity to develop critical thinking skills, assume leadership roles, and develop self-worth. They exhibited attitudes different from those of students with hospital diplomas. A 1962 comparison of hospital and university students found that those in the BSN program were more likely to value long-term careers, job satisfaction, autonomy, and financial security.[108] Another researcher, who interviewed California nursing students in the early 1960s, found those in four-year schools appeared more concerned with careers and continuing education than those in two and three year programs.[108]

The NLN Nurse Career-Pattern Study, which traced women who entered nursing school in 1962, found that the lives of college-educated nurses differed markedly from those of their hospital-trained peers. As early as five years after graduation fifty-three percent of BSNs held positions as educators, administrators, consultants, or researchers. Forty-one percent of hospital graduates held similar positions. Ten and fifteen years after graduation, R.N.s with college degrees were two to three times more likely to work in public health or nursing education, fields which paid well and afforded considerable autonomy. Thirty-one percent of both ADNs and BSNs had earned additional degrees, compared to twenty-six percent of DIs.[109]

Statistics on 1970s and 1980s graduates revealed similar patterns. Younger, married nurses, commited to their careers, increased their labor force participation after 1972.[110] As Lucie Young Kelly reported after her 1979 meeting with BSN students,

> All insisted that they were not going through a nursing education program to retire from the field when they graduated. Indeed a number were looking ahead to advanced education.... I found a similar attitude at the recent National Student Nurses' Association convention....[111]

Furthermore, those women who attended college during the cultural milieu of the 1960s acquired a willingness to question societal values and a militance about their own rights. Such attitudes were virtually unknow among hospital graduates. Professor Catherine Muldrow described the organizers of the Rutgers' boycott as "In tune with the times ... dynamic in their views and perspectives...." She also acknowledged their insistence upon controlling their own educations.[112] Over a decade later Lucie Young Kelly characterized 1960s college graduates as a "new breed" of nurse because of their campus activities.[113]

Higher education facilitated a revolution, which will be discussed further in Chapter 4. College graduates saw work as a salient part of their lives. They wanted salaries and benefits commensurate with their professional self-images. Education at community colleges and universities had taught them to ask questions about nursing's position in the American health care system. It had also empowered them to seek change. As Lucie Young Kelly warned *Nursing Outlook* readers in 1981,

> They learn to organize, they savor the strength of numbers; they taste success. While some become disillusioned or discouraged about changing the system, others simply bring their concepts of rights, authority, participation, and independence from the campus to their work setting. They are not easily cowed. They will fight for what they believe in — sooner or later.[114]

Endnotes

1. Alma S. Woolley, "My Lamp is Refueled," *AJN* 67 (August 1967): 1661-1664.

2. McLaughlin et al., *Changing Lives*, 33-34.

3. James Gilbert, *Another Chance: Postwar America, 1945-1968* (Philadelphia: Temple University Press, 1981), 21-24, 155, 215; Claudia Goldin, "The Meaning of College in The Lives of American Women: The Past One-Hundred Years," *National Bureau of Economic Research Working Paper Series* 4099 (June 1992): 5-6; Susan M.

Hartmann, *The Home Front and Beyond: American Women in the 1940s* (Boston: Twayne Publishers, 1982), 105-106; Barbara Miller Solomon, *In the Company of Educated Women: A History of Women and Higher Education in America* (New Haven: Yale University Press, 1985), 189-190, 198; Harold S. Wechsler, *The Qualified Student: A History of Selective College Admission in America* (New York: John Wiley and Sons, 1977), 259-263.

4. McLaughlin, et al., *Changing Lives*, 42-45, 48.

5. Evans, *Personal Politics*, 17-23, 98-101, 159-189; Goldin, "The Meaning of College," 28.

6. Esther Lucille Brown, "Professional Education for the Nursing of the Future," *AJN* 47 (December 1947): 821.

7. Rita Sinkevitch, "A Director of Nursing Speaks on Education," *The Pennsylvania Nurse* 22 (January 1967): 7.

8. Barbara G. Schutt, "More Than Two Hands," *AJN* 61 (July 1961): 43.

9. Schutt, "More Than Two Hands," 43.

10. Melosh, *"The Physician's Hand,"* 190.

11. Lulu Wolf Hassenplug, "Preparation of the Nurse Practitioner," *Journal of Nursing Education* 4 (January 1965): 34; Robert K. Merton, "Relations Between Registered Nurses and Licensed Practical Nurses: Status-Orientation in Nursing," *AJN* 62 (October 1962): 73; Irene Murchison, "A Four-Year Basic Collegiate Program," *AJN* 52 (April 1952): 483; Jeannette V. White, "Accelerated Evolution," *AJN* 49 (September 1949): 543.

12. Marion Sheahan, "The Health Needs of the Nation," *Nursing Outlook* 1 (March 1953): 156.

13. Agnes Gelinas, "Increasing the Number of Qualified Teachers," *AJN* 51 (August 1951): 528.

14. Kalisch and Kalisch, *Advance of Nursing*, 659.

15. Robert K. Merton, "The Search for Professional Status," *AJN* 60 (May 1960): 663.

16. Loretta E. Heidgerken, "About a Philosophy of Education," *Nursing Outlook* 17 (April 1969): 42.

17. Sister Virginia Kingsbury, "Educational Programs Will Be Broader," *AJN* 62 (December 1962): 85.

18. Agnes Gelinas, "Our Basic Educational Programs," *AJN* 49 (January 1949): 49.

19. Mary M. Roberts, "Our Profession and Our Government," *AJN* 49 (March 1949): 130.

20. Edith P. Lewis, "Nurses for a Growing Nation," *AJN* 57 (June 1957): 721; "Professional Nursing School Admissions Decline in 1956," *AJN* 57 (August 1957): 1006.

21. Hildegard E. Peplau, "Nurse-Doctor Relationships," *Nursing Forum* 51, no. 1 (1966): 74.

22. Margaret Brown Harty, "Trends in Nursing Education," *AJN* 68 (April 1968): 771.

23. Gilbert, *Another Chance*, 20-22; Goldin, "The Meaning of College," 5-6; Hartmann, *The Home Front and Beyond*, 105-106.

24. Gilbert, *Another Chance*, 155, 215-218.

25. ANA, *Facts, 1962-1963*, 102; Kalisch and Kalisch, *Advance of Nursing*, 590, 644; Edith S. Oshin, "How to Get Help For Your Education," *RN* 24 (November 1961): 44-51.

26. Kalisch and Kalisch, *Advance of Nursing*, 664, 679, 697-698; M. Gaie Rubenfeld et al., "The Nurse Training Act: Yesterday, Today, and...," *AJN* 81 (June 1981): 1202; Jessie M. Scott, "Federal Support for Nursing Education, 1964 to 1972," *AJN* 72 (October 1972): 1857-1858.

27. ANA, *Facts, 1969*, 120.

28. Kalisch and Kalisch, *Advance of Nursing*, 698; Beatrice M. Shriver, et al., "Follow-Up on Mental Health Trainees," *AJN* 67 (December 1967): 2572.

29. Win Kelley and Leslie Wilbur, *Teaching in The Community Junior College* (New York: Appleton-Century-Crofts, 1970), 6-11.

30. Kelley and Wilbur, *The Community Junior College*, 11-12; Dale Tillery and William L. Deegan, "The Evolution of Two-Year Colleges Through Four Generations," in *Renewing the American Community College*, ed. William L. Deegan, Dale Tillery and Associates (San Francisco: Jossey-Bass Publishers, 1985), 6-8.

31. Kelley and Wilbur, *The Community Junior College*, 12-14; Tillery and Deegan, "The Evolution of Two-Year Colleges," 9-13.

32. Kelley and Wilbur, *The Community Junior College*, 14.

33. Tillery and Deegan, "The Evolution of Two-Year Colleges," 4.

34. Georgeen H. DeChow, "The Development of an Associate Degree Nursing Program," *Journal of Nursing Education* 1 (September 1962): 35-36; Rosemarie Rizzo Parse, "The Advantages of the Associate Degree Program," *Journal of Nursing Education* 6 (August 1967): 17.

35. Mildred L. Montag, "Technical Education in Nursing?" *AJN* 63 (May 1963): 100-103.

36. ANA, "Education For Nursing," *AJN* 65 (December 1965): 106.

37. Shirley H. Fondiller, *The Entry Dilemma: The National League for Nursing and the Higher Education Movement, 1952-1972, With an Epilogue to 1983*, 2nd ed. (New York: National League for Nursing, 1983), 30; "National League For Nursing 1965 Convention," *Nursing Outlook* 13 (June 1965):36; "One Resolution is Revised at Final Business Meeting, *NLN News*, 7 May 1965, 13; "Resolutions Voted Friday," *NLN News*, 7 May 1965, 13.

38. ANA, "Education For Nursing," 107-108.

39. Susan Rimby Leighow, "Backrubs vs. Bach: Nursing and the Entry-Into-Practice Debate" (paper presented at the annual meeting of the History of Education Society, Atlanta, Ga., November 3, 1990).

40. Katherine E. Hillsmith, "From RN to BSN: Student Perceptions," *Nursing Outlook* 26 (February 1978): 98, 100.

41. Subject #1, interview by author, telephone, 5 June 1989; Subject #4, interview by author, 8 June 1989, Pittsburgh, Pennsylvania.

42. "American Nurses Association Convention, '80," *AJN* 80 (July 1980): 1321, 1328; "Eight Resolutions Win Approval After Hearings," *Nursing Outlook* 29 (July 1981): 391; Walter L. Johnson, "Educational Preparation for Nursing - 1974," *Nursing Outlook* 23 (September 1975): 582.

43. Subject #15, interview by author, tape recording, 7 July 1989, Doylestown, Pennsylvania.

44. Subject # 18, interview by author, 26 July 1989, Hershey, Pennsylvania.

45. Walter L. Johnson, "Educational Preparation - 1977," *Nursing Outlook* 25 (September 1978): 569.

46. "NLN Predicts Most Growth in Nursing School Graduations," *AJN* 84 (June 1984): 828; "Nursing Enrollments, Applications Fall Again; Closures Seen, But Some Schools Hold Their Own," *AJN* 86 (October 1986): 1178; "Schools Alarmed By Downturn In Applications; 'Pools Down In Quantity And Quality,' Some Say," *AJN* 85 (November 1985): 1292, 1299-1300; "Slack Economy Spurs Part-Time, RN Enrollments in BSN Programs," *AJN* 82 (August 1982):1194.

47. ANA, *Facts About Nursing, 1954* (New York: ANA, 1954), 18.

48. ANA, *Facts, 1964*, 10; ANA, *Facts, '72-'73*, 10.

49. ANA, *Facts, '80-'81*, 14; ANA, *Facts, '82-83*, 18.

50. Subject #5, interview by author, 9 June 1989, Pittsburgh, Pennsylvania.

51. Woolley, "My Lamp is Refueled," 1663-1664.

52. Elizabeth M. Maupin, "About Education for the Young at Heart," *Nursing Outlook* 15 (September 1967): 60.

53. Kathryn M. Lewis, "Back to School," *AJN* 73 (April 1973): 677.

54. Norma J. Melcom, "Letters," *AJN* 67 (August 1967): 1624.

55. Subjects #13 and #14, interview by author, tape recording, 28 June 1989, Ashland, Pennsylvania.

56. Susan L. Jones and Paul K. Jones, "Nursing Student Definitions of the 'Real Nurse,'" *Journal of Nursing Education* 16 (April 1977): 18; Louisa M. Murray and Donald R. Morris, "Professional Autonomy among Senior Nursing Students in Diploma, Associate Degree, and Baccalaureate Nursing Programs," *Nursing Research* 31 (September/October 1982): 313.

57. Subject #4.

58. Subject #1.

59. Subject #6, interview by author, 9 June, 1989, Pittsburgh, Pennsylvania.

60. Fourteen Authors, "The Professional Care and Treatment of Nurses," *Nursing Forum* 1 (Summer 1962): 85.

61. Peplau, "Nurse-Doctor Relationships," 72.

62. Nancy Carothers, "Letters," *AJN* 68 (October 1968): 2115.

63. Subject #23, interview by author, tape recording, 22 October 1989, Pittsburgh, Pennsylvania.

64. Norma K. Grand, "Our Readers Say," *Nursing Outlook* 14 (May 1966): 26.

65. Subject #2, interview by author, tape recording, 7 June 1989, Pittsburgh, Pennsylvania; Subject #3, tape recording, interview by author, 7 June 1989, Mars, Pennsylvania.

66. Subject #23.

67. Peplau, "Nurse-Doctor Relationships," 72.

68. Subject #22, interview by author, tape recording, 28 September 1989, Harrisburg, Pennsylvania.

69. Subject #3.

70. Subject #13.

71. Subject #5.

72. Lewis, "Back to School," 677; Subject #3; Subject #11, interview by author, 23 June 1989, Norristown, Pennsylvania.

73. Subject #18.

74. Edith P. Lewis, "Testimonial," *Nursing Outlook* 24 (February 1976): 83.

75. Yvonne Kemp, "Our Readers Say," *Nursing Outlook* 23 (September 1975): 538.

76. Subject #15.

77. Subject #18.

78. Subject #25, interview by author, tape recording, 23 October 1989, Pittsburgh, Pennsylvania.

79. Lucie Young Kelly, "Goodbye, Appliance Nurse," *Nursing Outlook* 27 (June 1979): 432.

80. Pamela A. Baj, "Demographic Characteristics of RN and Generic Students: Implications for Curriculum," *Journal of Nursing Education* 24 (June 1985): 232-234; Gortner, "Nursing Majors," 127; Hillsmith, "From R.N. to BSN," 99; Joan E. King, "A Comparative Study of Adult Developmental Patterns of RN and Generic Students in a Baccalaureate Nursing Program," *Journal of Nursing Education* 25 (November 1986): 368; Knopf, *Fifteen Years After Graduation*, 48; Frances L. Portnoy, "RN Students Analyze Their Experiences," *Nursing Outlook* 28 (February 1980): 112; Marcia J. Swanson, "Baccalaureate Nursing Education: Students' Perceptions of Roles, Effort, and Performance," *Journal of Nursing Education* 26 (November 1987): 381.

81. Woolley, "My Lamp Is Refueled," 1663.

82. Louise Malarkey, "The Older Student - stress or success on campus," *Journal of Nursing Education* 18 (February 1979): 18.

83. Myra S. Wilson, "Letters," *AJN* 69 (December 1969): 2592.

84. Lewis, "Back to School," 677.

85. Woolley, "My Lamp Is Refueled," 1664.

86. Todd Gitlin, *The Sixties: Years of Hope, Days of Rage* (New York: Bantam Books, 1987); James Miller, *"Democracy Is In The Streets:" From Port Huron To The Siege Of Chicago* (New York: Simon and Schuster, 1987).

87. Subject #1.

88. Subject #2.

89. Subject #15.

90. Dorothy W. Smith, "Views of a Faculty Member," *Nursing Forum* 8, no. 2 (1969): 138.

91. Patricia Bercik, "Views of a Senior Student," *Nursing Forum* 8, no. 2 (1969): 127-129.

92. Alice Lee Murray, "Our Readers Say," *Nursing Outlook* 18 (February 1970): 14.

93. Jean Markley, "Letters," *AJN* 70 (November 1970): 2334.

94. Ruth B. Freeman, "Practice as Protest," *AJN* 71 (May 1971): 919-921.

95. Tongee Jeu and Jane Raulston, "A Community Need - Nursing and Medical Students Respond," *Nursing Outlook* 18 (March 1970): 28-30.

96. "Students Testify On Health Care Crisis," *AJN* 71 (April 1971): 653.

97. "The Dallas Convention," *AJN* 71 (June 1971): 1176; "NSNA Convention," *Nursing Outlook* 18 (June 1970): 50-51; "NSNA 1970 Convention," *AJN* 70 (June 1970): 1311; "NSNA Convention - 1972" *Nursing Outlook* 20 (June 1972): 404; "NSNA - Past, Present, And Future," *Nursing Outlook* 18 (June 1970): 27; "Students Rap And Act," *Nursing Outlook* 19 (June 1971): 407-409.

98. Edith Patton Lewis, "Student Responsibility?" *Nursing Outlook* 17 (March 1969): 17.

99. Teresa Campbell and Sue Parsell, "Campus in Turmoil," *Nursing Outlook* 17 (June 1969): 78-79; Joanne Meaney, Christina Flanagan, and Kathy Horvath, "Views of Three Junior Students," *Nursing Forum* 8, no. 2 (1969): 12.

100. "Students to Hold Teach-In on Environment," *AJN* 70 (June 1970): 1179.

101. "Nursing Students Share In Campus Peace Observances," *AJN* 70 (June 1970): 1179.

102. Lewis, "Student Responsibility?" 17.

103. Lewis, "Student Responsibility?" 17; Cecil A. Ryder, Jr. and Fay O. Wilson, "The Power of Positive Student Action," *Nursing Outlook* 17 (March 1969): 18-19.

104. "The Dallas Conventions," *AJN* 71 (June 1971): 1176-1178; "NSNA Convention - 1972," *Nursing Outlook* 20 (June 1972): 404; "Students Rap And Act," 408-409.

105. Meaney, Flanagan, and Horvath, "Three Junior Students," 122-126; Catherine Muldrow, "Now It's Students of Nursing," *AJN* 69 (June 1969): 1252-1253.

106. Meaney, Flanagan, and Horvath, "Three Junior Students," 123-124.

107. Gortner, "Nursing Majors," 126-127.

108. Laura C. Dustan, "Characteristics Of Students in Three Types Of Nursing Education Programs," *Nursing Research* 13 (Spring 1964): 166.

109. Knopf, *Fifteen Years After Graduation* 18, 40, 46; NLN, "Nurse Career-Pattern Study: Baccalaureate Degree Nurses Ten Years After Graduation," *Hospital Topics* 57 (May/June 1979): 6.

110. Evelyn Moses and Aleda Roth, "Nursepower: What statistics tell us about the nation's nurses," *AJN* 79 (October 1979): 1746; Evelyn Moses, "Nurses Today - A Statistical Portrait," *AJN* 82 (March 1982): 448.

111. Kelly, "Goodbye, Appliance Nurse," 432.

112. Muldrow, "Now It's Students of Nursing," 1252.

113. Lucie Young Kelly, "The New Breed," *Nursing Outlook* 29 (July 1981): 440.

114. Kelley, "The New Breed," 440.

CHAPTER 4:

Connecting the "Nurses' Question and the Women's Question:" Registered Nurses and Feminism

In June 1982 the American Nurses Association held its biennial convention in Washington, D.C. On the 28th, amid applause and cheers, the House of Delegates unanimously passed a resolution endorsing the dying ERA. Two days later the delegates suspended their business meeting and joined an Equal Rights Amendment rally in Lafayette Park. Thousands of nurses carried signs and chanted slogans. ANA Directors, Eunice Cole and Carol Spengler, joined National Organization of Women (NOW) president, Eleanor Smeal, on the podium. On June 30 the ANA also sent a letter to ERA opponent, Phyllis Schafly. Here the association reaffirmed its commitment to the Amendment, as the period for ratification drew to a close.[1]

Scenes such as the one described above occurred frequently in the 1960s, 1970s, and early 1980s. During these years women increasingly demanded full equality. The feminist movement, which had floundered after the woman suffrage victory in 1919, saw a new resurgence. The demographic and social trends discussed earlier had significant roles in feminism's rebirth. For over two decades these forces led Americans to reconsider women's issues. Female professionals pressured John Kennedy into convening a Presidential Commission on the Status of Women in 1961. As the Commission uncovered evidence of widespread discrimination, these women lobbied for passage of the Equal Pay Act of 1963 and Title VII of the 1964 Civil Rights Act. During these same years the media examined the lives of college-educated women who had forgone careers for early marriage and motherhood. Betty Friedan's 1963 polemic, *The Feminine Mystique*, made the "trapped housewife" a

national problem. By mid-decade professional women created organizations such as NOW and the Women's Equity Action League
(WEAL).[2] The political and cultural ferment of the late 1960s and early
1970s gave these activists the opportunity to build coalitions in the wider
society.[3]

During these same years the baby boom generation also reached
adulthood. Their behavior had significant consequences for both American society and the women's movement. Younger college graduates,
for both financial and professional reasons, stayed in the work force
after marriage and motherhood. In 1960 roughly 17.5 percent of married women, aged 25-34 with children under 6 years old, worked outside the home. Ten years later the proportion was almost 30. By 1980
the figure was 45 percent. That year the ratio of labor force participation for married women with preschoolers to married childless women
was .98.[4]

Prolonged labor force participation enabled young women to
establish familes differently than their mothers had. Career-minded
baby boomers delayed matrimony. Median age at first marriage
began to climb in the early 1960s. It reached 24.0 for males and 22.1
for females in 1981. The annual marriage rate for that year was
slightly over 100 per 1,000 unmarried females, down significantly
from the 1950s' totals of 150-167. The number of divorces also rose
as economic independence allowed women to dissolve unhappy
unions. By 1980 the annual divorce rate was 22 per 1,000 married
females. As baby boomers concentrated on their jobs, they also post-
poned child-bearing and had fewer children. The fertility rate had
already decreased from a high of 3.7 in 1957 to roughly 3.5 in 1962.
Five years later it dropped to 2.5. By 1982 the fertility rate was
2.0, lower than it had been during the Great Depression.[5] Smaller
families gave women even more freedom and opportunity. Skilled,
well-educated, freed somewhat from traditional family constraints,
they adopted nontraditional attitudes about gender roles and
women's rights.[6] They assumed their equality with men, expected
fair treatment, and did not see themselves primarily as wives and
mothers.

At the same time, the social movements of the 1960s affected baby
boomers. Participation in civil rights struggles, for example, taught
young, college women the language of racism. They later used this
language to explain sex discrimination. The civil rights and student
movements also gave them alternative visions to the status quo. Pro-

testing segregation or the Vietnam War schooled them in the tactics of activism.[7]

These women — older professionals and the baby boomers — contributed different elements to the reborn feminist movement. The former group, disgusted with the discrimination they'd faced in the work place, wanted equal opportunities and rights in employment and politics. Their baby boomer counterparts were upset over sexism in groups such as SNCC and the SDS, and frustrated with traditional marriage. They hoped to end the sexual exploitation of women and forge new kinds of relationships and leadership styles. These younger feminists looked to transform the private as well as the public sphere.[8]

This divergence in experiences and goals created a movement composed, as Nancy F. Cott suggests, of several strands. One strand relied on a class-based, socialist anaylsis and set of tactics. The radical feminist strand, embodied by the activists of SNCC and SDS, saw gender as more significant than class. These young females formed consciousness-raising groups, fought patriarchal marriages and the sexual double standard, and talked about "women's liberation." For them, legalized abortion and accessible daycare were fundamental issues. A liberal feminist strand, composed of female professionals, focused on guaranteeing equal treatment for women within the existing democratic framework. They concentrated on utilizing affirmative action and fighting discrimination through the court system. Liberal feminists made ratification of the Equal Rights Amendment their number one priority. By the early 1970s these latter two strands blurred somewhat. Women's liberation became a more mainstream movement. NOW chapters, for example, championed reproductive rights and ran consciousness-raising sessions. Radical feminists supported the ERA. [9]

Whatever the strand feminism, particularly in the late 1960s and early 1970s, was characterized as a middle class phenomenon. Equality at work and home seemed to enhance the lives of the affluent, college-educated, white women involved in the movement. Working class females and women of color saw few benefits in feminism, particularly the largely symbolic ERA. Even the Coalition of Labor Union Women, formed in 1974, had more success in promoting females into union leadership positions than in solving the problems of the working class.[10]

Within this context nurses discovered and identified with feminism. Increased labor force participation and college education led professionally-minded nurses to reconsider old problems. Encouraged by their college and workplace experiences, influenced by the social upheaval of the 1960s, a minority of nurses became aware of sex discrimination. They recognized the truth of what Lavinia Dock had stated in 1907. Nurses' attempts to improve their working conditions and personal lives were connected with the larger question of women's equality.[11] Inadequate salaries, lack of autonomy, and the difficulty of juggling work and family suddenly looked different, examined under a feminist lens.

These nurses developed a feminist consciousness. They supported sexual equality and opposed the sex hierarchy in American society. They believed that women's condition was socially constructed and that, because of their socialization, females shared common ground. Feminist R.N.s also sought to mobilize other women in support of change.[12] Throughout the 1970s and early 1980s they utilized the nursing press, professional associations, and other venues to educate their peers. They forced the ANA to re-evaluate its long-standing opposition to the ERA.[13] They formed feminist nursing organizations, both as support groups and as agents for change. As was true in the larger society, specific groups of nurses, rather than a cross section of the profession, embraced the women's movement. Nursing also contained several different strands of feminism. Thus, studying nursing illuminates the forces which attracted women to the movement as well as the goals and tactics of its various strands.

Significant trends in the late 1960s and 1970s laid the foundation for feminist nursing activity. One factor concerned the employment of younger, married women. Wives and mothers had become an increasingly large segment of the nursing labor force since the mid-1950s. By 1966 they comprised two-thirds of employed R.N.s.[14] These women were, however, mostly over the age of forty-five. After 1966 younger nurses increased their labor force participation. In 1962 and 1966 one-half of all married nurses in their thirties and two-thirds of those in their forties were employed. By 1972 the proportions had increased to sixty-six and seventy-two percent.[15] During the rest of the decade younger married women's employment continued to rise (See Figure 10). At the same time working nurses' ages declined. After reaching a high of 40.3 in 1966, their median age decreased to 39.4 in 1972. In 1977 and 1980 the figures dropped to 37.7 and 36.3. By the close of the 1970s, 69.2 percent of employed R.N.s were under forty-five years of age.[16] Fifty-eight percent of nurses with infants and sixty-four percent of those with preschoolers worked outside the home.[17] R.N.s with children under thirteen years of age had employment rates nineteen percent higher than elementary school teachers and twenty-seven percent higher than women in other feminized professions.[18]

FIGURE 10: PERCENTAGE OF MARRIED NURSES IN THE LABOR FORCE IN EACH AGE COHORT, 1972-1980[a]

	20-24	25-29	30-34	35-39	40-44	45-49	50-54
1972	90	76	66	67	71	73	74
1977	93	83	70	70	74	72	72
1980	95	87	82	76	79	80	75

a.   *Source:* ANA, *Facts, 86-87,* 12.

The economic crisis of the 1970s was one factor which propelled younger women into the labor force. After nearly three decades of steady growth, the American economy began to founder. Inflation rates, which had been about two percent annually in the 1950s and 1960s, began to climb after 1972.[19] By mid-decade they had reached eight percent. Betwen 1977 and 1980 inflation rates approached yearly levels of eleven to fourteen percent.[20] At the same time the decline of basic industries such as steel, automobiles, and coal led to high, chronic unemployment and underemployment in sections of the Northeast and Midwest.[21] Baby-boom couples, raised in postwar affluence and concerned with establishing financial security, seemed particularly vulnerable to the shaky economy.[22] Younger wives felt they could not leave the labor force, even temporarily. Their paychecks were critical for family survival. In 1972, for example, women contributed twenty-eight percent of the family income if they worked part-time and forty percent if they worked full-time.[23]

Nurses, like other American women, responded to this economic dislocation. Financial need proved to be a major influence on their employment decisions during the 1970s. One woman, a twenty-seven year old mother of four from northeastern Pennsylvania, returned to part-time work because of rising inflation. Many of her peers worked full-time because their coal-miner husbands were unemployed.[24] A suburban Philadelphia mother of six also returned to nursing at the age of forty-three. Her motive was to preserve her family's middle class standard of living.[25] Inflation and unemployment thus accomplished what the professional associations had not been able to do. These economic forces at least temporarily ameliorated the nursing shortage. By the early 1980s hospital vacancy rates and turnover had declined. Employers attributed this to nurses' economic need.[26]

Professional commitment, particularly among college graduates, also caused young mothers to work. As Lucie Young Kelly had observed, these women were more likely to perceive nursing as a career and less likely to retire after marriage and motherhood.[27] Those who invested heavily in their educations and enjoyed nursing often adjusted poorly to full-time homemaking. One BSN recalled feeling professionally and socially isolated, despite her delight with her infant son. She returned to nursing nine months later as a hospital shift supervisor, even though she had promised the adoption agency that she would not work.[28] A public health nurse, who had quit her job to give birth, experienced "separation anxiety," "periods of depression," and "feelings of despair."[29] Other young mothers, aware of their intrinsic needs, never left the labor force. One R.N, who had both graduated from college and married in 1964, continued working after her daughter's birth two years later.[30] An MSN, who confided she would "drink or be in Harrisburg State [the local mental hospital]" if she wasn't employed, took short maternity leaves in the early 1970s during her two pregnancies. She returned to her job within a few months of each child's birth.[31]

As these younger nurses remained in the work force, they experienced considerable frustration. Salaries, acceptable to an older generation of part-time middle class homemakers, looked increasingly inadequate. College graduates, in particular, felt underpaid and overworked when they compared themselves to other professionals.[32] During the mid- and late 1960s they complained bitterly about wages in the nursing press. One BSN fumed in 1967 that her take-home pay was less than that of waitresses and hairdressers.[33] Another lamented, "What has happened to the image of nursing when truck drivers and unskilled laborers earn more than nurses?"[34]

Rising inflation choked already deficient salaries. In 1973 and 1974 the professional associations reported that nurses' wages lagged behind inflation.[35] *Nursing* magazine reported that salaries rose 27 percent betwen 1974 and 1977. Nurses, however, made "very little real wage gain" because the inflation rate climbed 25.8 percent.[36] By 1979 nurses actually lost ground when wages increased 2.8 percent less than the 1977-1979 cost of living.[37] R.N.s keenly felt the twin effects of high inflation and stagnant wages. One mother complained in 1972 that she could not "pay the mortgage, feed empty stomachs, educate children, or find a housekeeper" on her salary.[38] Two years later another reported, "By the time I buy my uniforms, pay for my meals, pay the baby-sitter, and add in transportation costs, I earn less than 50 cents an hour."[39]

Nurses also complained more about the lack of autonomy and physicians' attitudes. R.N.s increasingly asserted their right to function as full-fledged professionals. Doctors resisted deviations from the traditional, handmaiden role. In 1962 New Jersey and New York nurses fretted that

> Many a doctor stil measures a "good nurse" by how well she accommodates herself to his unscheduled hospital visits, to his medical and treatment orders, to his professional need for nursing assistance, and to his personal need to feel the "boss" in any professional situation. In the judgment of some, be they intern, resident, or attending physician, diplomacy and tact in handling a doctor's most pronounced quality - his independence - is the most important skill a nurse can possess. Secondary to this is her techincal and professional competence.[40]

Four years later a Michigan woman voiced similar criticism about "The 'sacred cow' of hospital management, which expects servile obedience and submission...."[41] Nurses were not the only ones to voice concern. Leonard Stein, a psychiatrist writing for the *AJN* in 1968, admitted that physicians were intolerant of outspoken nurses and threatened by attempts at collegiality. Stein referred to the traditional doctor-nurse relationship as both a "game" and "a transactional neurosis."[42]

Two incidents, which occurred at the AMA's 1965 and 1966 conventions, illustrate the friction between M.D.s and R.N.s at mid-decade. In 1965 the association publicized a program session entitled "Nurse-Physician Communications" and invited nurses to attend. In its convention coverage, the *AJN* noted that less than a dozen medical doctors came to the presentation.[43] One year later, at a similar program, only 36 of 500 audience members were physicians. These M.D.s spent most of the meeting criticizing the ANA Position Paper on Education.[44] Ingeborg Mauksch, a nursing educator who attended the 1966 session, likened the poor physician attendance to "dinner guests being served in the absence of their host." She also wrote, angrily, that "the sense of paternalism" on the part of doctors offended nurses who had "attended the program in good faith."[45]

Complaints about high-handed physicians intensified in the early 1970s. One R.N. indignantly related an incident in which M.D.s reprimanded hospital nurses for requesting consultations. "Consultation forms were for medical staff use only."[46] Another repeating a conversation with a physician co-worker complained,

> If a nurse on his staff questions a ridiculous medical order she is liable to be dubbed arrogant, intolerant, contentious, argumentative, or disrespectful of superior authority.
>
> Playing subservient is still the only way to play the game in many places.[47]

College-educated nurses found it particularly difficult to forge mutually respectful relationships with doctors. Two Pittsburgh BSNs, who worked in nursing administration during the early 1970s, recalled that many M.D.s were rude and abusive. R.N.s achieved success only when they "played male physician games" and acted subservient.[48]

A 1974 *Nursing* survey found these incidents to be the rule rather than the exception. Sixty-three percent of the participating nurses "often," "frequently," or "almost always" felt "used as a servant by a doctor." Several respondents related incidents of extreme acrimony between the two groups. One described an incident in which she had made "the unpardonable error of questioning a medication dosage." Not surprisingly, she expressed disgust with "the-doctor-is-always-right mentality." A staff nurse in a large, teaching hospital characterized M.D.s as "downright obnoxious." College-educated, younger R.N.s had the most complaints about physicians.[49]

Besides low salaries and lack of respect, young nurses were distressed over the daily strain of juggling work and family. The on-site daycare facilities established in the 1950s were inadequate a decade later as more mothers engaged in paid labor. In the mid-to-late 1960s and 1970s decent childcare was both difficult to find and expensive. In 1963 ANA lobbyist, Julia Thompson, testified before a federal committee that only half of the American children who needed daycare had access to licensed facilities.[50] Throughout the decade the association also urged Congress to liberalize childcare tax deductions.[51] Scheduling also became a more complicated issue. During the 1950s and early 1960s nurses had gratefully worked continuous weekends when their husbands were at home. Divorced women, however, had no weekend coverage. Baby-boomers, who were willing to use daycare facilities, wanted "to work the way the rest of the world works."[52] As one Brooklyn nurse stated,

> A mother can't work every weekend. Kareem [her son] is two years old. What happens to him when I work five weekends in a row?[53]

Young mothers found their concerns received little if any recognition. Discussions about publicly funded childcare provoked hostility. In some communities opposition hampered efforts to organize even private facilities. A board member for a nurses' daycare center pointed out in 1972,

> How has the center been received in our town? Not all are equally enthusiastic and some even regard day care for children as downright evil.[54]

The lack of appropriate childcare made the juggling act more difficult. A psychiatric nurse, forced back to work for economic reasons in the 1960s, recalled that problems with daycare made her feel "really shitty" about leaving her son.[55] Disapproving or uncooperative family members, neighbors, and even employers made already harried women feel guilty. One young mother, for example, returned to nursing in 1970 after her divorce. She experienced considerable antagonism in her Italian-American community.[56] Household duties compounded the stress. Employed nurses generally assumed all, or the majority, of domestic chores. As a hospital staff nurse remarked, her co-workers "supported the family because the mines were shut down, but still carried on all the home responsibilities because that was a woman's job."[57]

Nurses' growing frustration over salaries, autonomy, and the demands of balancing career and family coincided with the upheaval of the 1960s. Licensed R.N.s, as well as college students, witnessed the era's social movements. Even the normally conservative nursing press showed interest in activism. Throughout the late 1960s and early 1970s the major journals reported and offered commentary on pressing societal issues. The *AJN* was particularly conscientious about covering contemporary topics during Barbara Schutt's editorship from 1959 to 1971. Following the assassination of Martin Luther King in 1968, and again in 1969, Schutt wrote sensitive editorials about discrimination in nursing schools and hospitals.[58] Over the next two years she commented on the deaths of Kent State University students and reported on the founding of the Committee on Nursing in a Society in Crisis. Schutt also encouraged *AJN* staff to cover political and social topics and urged nurses to promote change.[59] In 1968, for example, she called for R.N.s to challenge the medical "Establishment" and "formulate a climate for decent health care, representing the interests of patients...."[60] In 1970 she suggested public health nurses investigate and end malnutrition.[61] Such coverage both facilitated nurses' political awareness and encouraged them to debate contemporary subjects. By the early 1970s readers increasingly filled the *AJN's* pages with letters on social issues.[62]

Urged on by the professional press and leadership, nurses participated in the movements of the 1960s and 1970s.[63] ANA officers created an Affirmative Action Taskforce and formed coalitions with civil rights groups.[64] During the mid-1960s nurses participated in "Mississippi Summers" where they provided health care for both civil rights workers and local black families.[65] By the early 1970s R.N.s marched in anti-war rallies and gave emergency treatment to sick and injured protestors.[66] Nurses also involved themselves in poverty projects. In Portland, Oregon a group of NLN members co-sponsored a people's clinic with the local Black Panthers.[67] A Harrisburg, Pennsylvania nurse operated a storefront clinic which served transients and welfare recipients.[68] Activist Marion Moses worked with striking California migrant workers from 1968 through 1971. Moses managed a union-operated health facility, made home nursing visits, and developed the farm workers' Health and Welfare Plan.[69]

As nurses marched in rallies or worked in free clinics they gained political and leadership skills. The experiences of three Northern R.N.s, who spent a summer in Mississippi with the Medical Committee on Human Rights, is one such example. The visiting nurses performed their assigned duties of caring for patients and teaching health classes. They also met with local black community groups to discuss ways of gaining better treatment from the local health department. In the process they learned to mobilize people and translate their concerns into concrete actions. Hospital graduates, these R.N.s recognized the value of this hands-on experience. In an *AJN* article they observed, "Our formal nursing education did not quite equip us for this type of community work."[70] Marion Moses experienced a similar political education as she helped organize a grape boycott, raised funds for striking migrant workers, and interceded for patients with local hospitals and physicians.[71]

These nurses also learned to withstand criticism. Women who worked with civil rights activists or marched against the Vietnam War learned to face "danger, hostility, and harassment." In some cases they dealt with a "community [which] did not welcome our presence...."[72] They also came to identify with past nurse-radicals such as Lillian Wald and Lavinia Dock. As NLN official, Lucille Knopf, pointed out, "We were founded by women active in the suffragettes...."[73] Becoming comfortable with rebellion had important consequences for women who had worked in hierarchical settings and were accustomed to taking orders.[74]

This convergence of social rebellion with nurses' ever-growing dissatisfaction created a revolt of sorts within the profession. By the early

1970s a minority of R.N.s identified with the re-emerging women's movement. As was true in the larger society, nurse-feminists came primarily from two distinct groups. Employed nurses with college degrees, frustrated with low salaries and lack of respect, came to accept the movement's critique of male-dominated society. Many of these women worked in what were considered elite fields — nursing education and administration — or they had a clinical specialty. These nurses, well-educated and employed in relatively autonomous settings, traditionally exhibited less subservience than hospital staff.[75] At the same time baby boomers, socialized as professionals and schooled in campus activism, joined the nursing work force. These younger women entered practice with an awareness of the sex hierarchy and a determination to change the status quo. At this time class was less of a dividing line for feminist nurses. Public funding of nursing education, as discussed in Chapter 3, had enabled many working class women to enroll in collegiate programs.

Nurses learned of feminism in a variety of ways. The nursing press reported on the women's movement with increasing frequency. In 1963 assistant *AJN* editor, Gretchen Gerds, interviewed Esther Peterson, executive vice-chair of the President's Commission on the Status of Women.[76] In 1966 and 1967 the *Journal* carried information on Title VII and the Equal Employment Opportunity Commission.[77] By the early 1970s articles on topics such as sex discrimination, pertinent court decisions, and abortion appeared in almost every issue.[78]

Nurses learned about feminism from other sources as well. The print and television media focused increasing attention on the movement in the 1970s. Much of this coverage was negative in tone, concerned with sensationalized incidents such as bra-burnings. Yet the media aroused nurses' curiosity and interest.[79] Those inclined read more positive accounts in publications such as *Ms.* or attended NOW meetings.[80] Friends also spread feminism's message. Baby boomers discussed the women's movement during late-night dormitory bull sessions and at weekend college parties.[81] Three young R.N.s, who worked in a hospital emergency room in the 1970s, discussed feminism during lulls in the routine.[82]

By the early 1970s the frustrated nurses discussed above had developed a feminist consciousness. Nowhere was this more evident than in the professional press. Journals began to publish articles which analyzed nursing's problems from a feminist perspective. Authors exhorted their audiences to ally themselves with the women's movement.

The first series of consciousness-raising articles appeared in the *American Journal of Nursing* in February 1971. This issue featured three articles on both women's rights and the ERA. The editorial page contained a series of "Guest Opinions" written by nursing professors active in NOW and WEAL.[83] These editorials analyzed sexism's impact on American society and its implications for nursing. They suggested that nurses' problems stemmed from a sex hierarchy which deliberately socialized women into accepting inferior roles. Guest editors argued that American women were not physically or mentally inferior to men. The authors recognized, however, that females achieved less because of inferior educations, rigid gender stereotypes, and male domination.[84] Not content to simply define the problem, the guest editors called for nurses to join with other women in support of equal rights.[85] Both the February articles and the editorials also dealt specifically with sexism within nursing. In particular the authors argued that nurse-physician conflict was a function of sex discrimination. They blamed the problem on educational inequities and cultural attitudes about female subservience.[86]

Six months later a more detailed analysis appeared in the *AJN*. Tellingly entitled, "Sex Discrimination: Nursing's Most Pervasive Problem," author Virginia Cleland convincingly argued that sexism had a profound effect upon the profession. Cleland was a nursing educator who had successfully combined family life with a distinguished career. She had also recently initiated a sex discrimination complaint against her employer, Wayne State University. Cleland could thus speak first-hand about the link between female inequality and nursing. She admitted that she had only recently embraced feminism. In fact she dated her interest in the women's movement to 1970 when she joined a consciousness-raising group. As she read feminist literature,

> I begin to recognize how closely the entire social issue of equal rights for women actually relates to nursing. Today, there is no doubt in my mind that our most fundamental problem in nursing is that we are members of a woman's occupation in a male-dominated culture.[87]

Cleland blamed this male-dominated society for nurses' professional problems — low wages, poor benefits, the difficulties of combining work and family, lack of power. Like the SNCC and SDS activists described by historian Sara Evans, Cleland used the language of racism to describe R.N.'s plight. She likened the postion of nurses in the health care system to "the exploitation of Negroes in our culture." She also compared hospital nursing directors to "black principals in the separate Southern black school systems" and labeled nursing leaders as "female Uncle Toms." Cleland proposed to end sexism by providing women with equal access to higher education, fair wages and equitable benefits. She also called for the end of the sexual division of labor within the family.[88]

Readers' reactions in 1971 were primarily sympathetic. Responses to the *AJN's* February edition, for example, were positive. A NOW member wrote, "The February issue on equal rights for women was long overdue and most welcome."[89] Another nurse "applauded" the *Journal* for its coverage.[90] A periodical known for publishing diverse points of view, the *AJN* printed ten responses to Cleland's article, all of which were favorable. Many respondents seemed relieved that the issue of sexism in nursing had finally been addressed. In the words of one long-practicing nurse,

> Virginia Cleland has put down in black and white numerous things which have needed saying for years, but which one would hardly dare think, let alone verbalize.[91]

Consciousness-raising continued in both the *AJN* and *Nursing Outlook* over the course of the decade. Some articles, such as Wilma Scott Heide's "Nursing and Women's Liberation: A Parallel," spoke in general terms about sexism in society and nursing.[92] Authors such as nursing professor, Angela Barron McBride, criticized inequitable family relations.[93] Others more specifically targeted nursing's professional problems. Yale University faculty argued in 1972 that nurses failed to exhibit leadership skills. They blamed this on traditional educational practices which socialized students to be deferential and passive.[94] Feminist authors studied wage disparities between nursing and male-dominated professions. They argued that R.N.s' lower salaries reflected society's devaluation of women's work.[95] Nursing also analyzed its image. Women seemed particularly upset over media portrayals of R.N.s. One, writing in 1973, vigorously complained about television programs, movies, and novels which stereotyped nurses "in the handmaiden, social, or secretarial role." She decried the depiction of R.N.s "as frivolous or incompetent."[96] Other feminists scorned slogans such as "Love A Nurse" and complained about gender stereotypes in professional advertisements.[97]

These consciousness-raising pieces also dealt with physician-nurse relationships and the profession's struggle for autonomy. One of the earliest and most detailed discussions of this problem was nursing professor JoAnn Ashley's "About Power in Nursing." Published in the

October 1973 issue of *Nursing Outlook*, the article addressed nursing's inabilty to influence health care practices or control its own destiny. Ashley argued that the problem stemmed from medicine's domination of its sister profession. She described physicians as "medical men [who] view themselves as a ruling class." M.D.s believed "that nurses had to be intellectually and socially controlled" and "supported the view that nurses exist to serve physicians." The medical profession had successfully "undermined the confidence of nurses and their power to affect change...."[98] Ashley, a socialist feminist, argued from both a class and a gender framework. She even referred to R.N.s as "the trained nurse proletariat."[99] Two years later in "Nursing and Early Feminism," Ashley futher argued that negative working conditions, particularly low pay and long hours, were direct consequences of nurses' exploitation as women and workers.[100]

Numerous other authors expanded on this theme. A year after the publication of "About Power in Nursing," Yale professor Katherine Nuckolls wrote an article on the patriarchal health care system. She attributed this situation both to nurses' socialization as females and male doctors' hostility toward competent women.[101] In 1976 *Nursing Outlook* associate editor, Jeanne Fonesca, characterized nurses as "passive, submissive, obedient, wife-mothers" victimized by physicians' domination.[102] Four years later nursing educator, Gloria Smith, drew a parallel between medicine's control of nursing and white exploitation of African-Americans. Smith referred to the health care system as "the last plantation."[103] By the late 1970s and early 1980s nurses discussed strategies for resisting physician domination. They included such diverse tactics as collaborative practices, nursing registeries, feminist education courses, and assertiveness training.[104]

Consciousnes-raising occurred at professional conventions as well as through the nursing press. In 1974 the ANA featured convention sessions on "Women's Rights and the Nurse" and "Women Power." Speakers included Wilma Scott Heide, a nurse and past NOW president. Convention-goers learned about the Equal Rights Amendment, the problem of accessible childcare, and the need for more research on women's illnesses.[105] In 1975 the NLN sponsored a convention program entitled "Women *in* Power, Nurses *in* Power" at which speakers discussed the need for nurses to take on leadership roles.[106] At later conventions ANA and NLN delegates explored gender discrimination in the work place, nursing's public image, and nonsexist models of professional practice. These programs validated members' feelings of frustration and offered alternatives to the status quo.[107]

During the 1970s consciousness-raising also occurred in educational institutions. Faculty members incorporated feminist perspectives in nursing ethics classes or designed new courses dealing with women's issues.[108] Students also disseminated information to their teachers. One dean of nursing recalled attending a graduate student panel on nursing and the women's movement in the early 1970s. She was so struck by the accuracy of their analysis that she invited two of the panelists back to her office to continue the discussion.[109] Students raised each other's consciousness in classes and dormitories, as well as at social events.[110]

Like women in the larger society, nurses also met in small groups to discuss sex discrimination. In 1979 two clinical specialists, who led all nurse consciousness-raising groups, described their experiences in the *AJN*. Over a period of several months R.N.s met and discussed "the socially conditioned and automatic roles and responses of women." They analyzed "the stereotypes of wife, mother, single woman, career women, and women in general." By examining "issues that are basic to being female — sexism, anger, roles and role models, body image, rape, sexuality — group members became more aware of the reasons behind their behavior." They then became "freer to explore alternatives."[111]

This consciousness-raising enabled women to connect the nursing question and the women's question. It also led them to support the larger feminist cause. As ANA members became involved in the movement, the association participated in feminist rallies and conferences, testified on pertinent legislation, and allied itself with like-minded women's organizations.[112] During the 1970s and early 1980s the normally conservative ANA supported female political candidates. It publicly promoted women's equal access to education, employment, and health care.[113]

As nurses discovered and accepted feminism they confronted the movements two most critical issues — reproductive choice and the Equal Rights Amendment. The ANA approached abortion gingerly, even though several state affiliates took pro-choice positions.[114] A resolution passed at the 1968 convention called solely for an examination of present statutes. The delegates advocated "legal termination of pregnancy" only in cases where a mother's life was at risk, fetal anomalies were likely, or the pregnancy was a result of rape or incest.[115] As such it fell far short of the women's movement's position. Pro-life nurses, however, sharply criticized the ANA's moderate stance.[116] In an effort to accommodate members of diverse beliefs, the association uttered no further pronouncements in the 1970s and early 1980s. The NLN likewise stayed neutral, despite attempts by both pro-choice and pro-life members to force the issue at the 1981 convention.[117]

The professional associations did, however, reevaluate their longstanding opposition to the ERA. The ANA had feared the Amendment's passage would neutralize the protective legislation which had covered working women since the Progressive era.[118] At the 1954 convention Board member, Janet Geister, insisted that women needed these laws to protect their health and safety.[119] By the 1970s, however, feminist nurses perceived the issue differently. They saw themselves as full-fledged professionals, worked for a large part of their lifetimes, and supported families. From their perspective, women needed *equal* rather than special treatment under the law. The *AJN's* Thelma Schorr accurately described their position in a 1971 editorial. Schorr asserted that protective legislation had done little to solve the problems of American nurses.

> Oponents of the Amendment maintain that its passage will mean that women will not be protected from working long hours, night shifts, or while pregnant; that they will risk losing the financial support of their husbands or their alimony if divorced; and that they could be subject to the draft, among other things. Well, nurses have always had the dubious privilege of working nights and overtime; they have come close to being drafted several times and certainly would have been had they not responded in sufficient numbers to wartime needs. Many a nurse has put a husband through college and, with the law of supply and demand on her side, she has been granted maternity leave and often been permitted to work until the day of delivery.[120]

Feminists nurses also argued that the passage of ERA would equalize existing wage laws and make it easier for female workers, including R.N.s, to sue for sex discrimination.[121]

The ANA's Board of Directors reversed its opposition and voted to support the ERA in 1971.[122] Until 1982, when the ratification period ended, the association actively worked for the ERA's passage. Convention delegates issued frequent resolutions calling for the Amendment's ratification. Through the ANA's political action committtee, Nurses Coalition for Action in Politics (N-CAP), members lobbied legislators.[123] In 1978 the House of Delegates upheld a Board decision to hold association meetings only in ratified states.[124] R.N.s also marched, lobbied, and leafleted for the ERA through their state-level ANA affiliates.[125] The Illinois Nurses Association even refused to meet in its own, unratified state and held its 1979 convention in neighboring Wisconsin.[126] Although less involved than its sister organization, the NLN also took a stand on the Equal Rights Amendment. Delegates voted to support the ERA during the 1975 convention and to meet only in ratified states in 1977.[127]

Feminists nurses also formed groups outside the established professional associations. These organizations functioned as consciousness-raising vehicles and support networks. Their founders saw them as potential change agents, able to attack sexism more directly than the traditionally conservative ANA and NLN. These nursing groups also represented various strands of feminism. Studying two such groups, Nurses NOW and Cassandra, sheds further light on the goals and tactics of feminist R.N.s. It also helps define the similarities and differences among the several branches of the American women's movement.

Nurses NOW originated at the National Organization of Women's 1973 convention. During the meeting twenty-five nurses responded to a bulletin board notice and met to discuss their common problems.[128] They realized the need to approach the subject from both a feminist and a professional perspective. The women thus decided to form "task forces" solely for nurses in their home communities.[129] In 1974, these local groups were incorporated as Nurses NOW, NOW's first national occupational task force. By 1977 the organization had thirty-eight chapters.[130] Because a majority of the core group came from Pittsburgh, that city served as national headquarters. The Pittsburgh chapter thus became the driving force behind Nurses NOW. Its members published the national newsletter, coordinated fundraising and lobbying activities, and represented the organization at various professional functions.[131]

Like Nurses NOW, Cassandra members first met at a larger meeting. Twelve nurses, upset over the demise of the ERA, met to discuss future strategy at the 1982 ANA convention. They decided to form a distinctly feminist nursing organization. Casting about for a name, the women called their group Cassandra, after the mythological creature in one of Florence Nightingale's essays. According to Nightingale, Cassandra had the gift of prophecy, but was neither heard nor believed.[132] By publicizing in journals such as the *AJN* and *Ms.* and attending professional conventions, the orginal members forged ties with other feminist nurses.[133] By 1985 Cassandra had forty contact women living in twenty-seven states and Canada. While many of the local groups existed in liberal Northeastern and Midwestern cities, Cassandra also formed chapters in more conservative states such as Utah.[134]

Nurses NOW and Cassandra shared many goals — consciousness-raising among nurses, mobilizing R.N.s on relevant issues, and providing support for sister feminists.[135] The two groups were also similar in terms of age and occupational characteristics. Nurses NOW members were mostly college-educated baby boomers who worked in public health or the lower levels of hospital administration. Members had both middle and working class backgrounds.[136] Cassandra chapters contained college students and professors, administrators, and clinical specialists in areas such as public health and psychiatric nursing. One group included a nursing journal editor.[137] Both networks, then, were comprised of nursing's elite. Here, however, the similarities ended. Nurses NOW and Cassandra differed philosophically. They also adopted divergent leadership styles, causes, and tactics.

Although considered radicals by older, more traditional colleagues and supervisors, Nurses NOW members were actually liberal feminists.[138] One, for example, characterized herself as "never revolutionary, but always responsive to sexism."[139] These women focused on what they perceived as "manageable" problems such as salary and autonomy issues. Their ultimate goal was to gain equity with male health care professionals. They sought to affect change by both "empowering" other nurses and mobilizing existing organizations. In Pittsburgh, for example, a number of women from Nurses NOW joined the Pennsylvania Nurses Association and tried to instill feminist consciousness in its members.[140] They also attempted to organize collective bargaining units in several area hospitals.[141] In 1976 Nurses NOW held a conference on temporary nursing agencies. Here the organization publicized agencies' negative impact on patient care and nurses' working conditions.[142] For the most part, the group steered clear of issues which did not directly affect its members or were considered controversial. Pittsburgh Nurses NOW, for example, did not address daycare because few of its members had children.[143] It likewise shied away from abortion. After intial meetings with a gay nurses group in 1974, the chapter backed off. Support for people of diverse sexual orientations "created havoc back home."[144]

Cassandra, on the other hand, was unabashedly radical. It welcomed women with diverse sexual preferences and encouraged nurses to engage in "personal and professional revolutionary acts."[145]

Cassandra members were interested in transforming the entire health care system as well as empowering nurses. They supported a number of innovations such as natural remedies, woman-centered birthing practices, and female control over reproductive technologies.[146] Local Cassandra groups also involved themselves in larger women's issues. In 1984, for example, the Buffalo chapter sponsored Wilma Scott Heide's visit to the city's International Women's Day celebration. A year later Buffalo members participated, along with other women's groups, in a "Take Back the Night" march to protest violence against females.[147] Cassandra also promoted women's music, poetry, and bookstores.[148]

Nurses NOW and Cassandra differed in organizational structure. Nurses NOW had an orderly configuration, complete with a national coordinator and annual dues. Local chapters, such as the one in Pittsburgh, also had formal offices.[149] Cassandra, on the other hand, eschewed formal organizational structures. Like the women involved in SNCC and the SDS, they wanted to transform "patriarchal" leadership styles. Members thus opted for a casual framework which they hoped would be more democratic. Cassandra had no national officers per se. It asked members for an unspecified "financial contribution" instead of charging flat, yearly dues.[150] Local chapters bypassed organizational language and parliamentary procedure. They referred to their groups as "webs" and their members as "websters." Websters led meetings on a rotating basis. Discussions continued until consensus was reached. Many webs "passed the hat" for donations.[151] Although the national body incorporated in 1985 for legal reasons, decision-making remained democratic and decentralized.[152]

The two groups also mobilized members differently. Their reactions to the ERA are a case in point. Both networks expressed support for the Amendment. As had been true earlier with suffrage, the Equal Rights Amendment was ambiguous enough to unite women with otherwise divergent values.[153] But if nurses' responses are in any way representative, liberal and radical feminists approached ratification differently. Nurses NOW, for example, urged members to write letters to elected officials and boycott companies headquartered in unratified states.[154] Cassandra encouraged websters to develop their own, individualistic approaches. In the words of one columnist,

> We receive many inquiries about our plan of action on the ERA or political action of other types. Cassandra has no structure to deal with these issues at this time.

Instead, she advocated "personal" and "creative solutions."[155] Such action could take many forms. In 1982, for example, one *Newsjournal* correspondent protested the demise of ERA by climbing over the White House fence and later pouring blood on a replica of the U.S. Constitution.[156]

Whether liberal or radical, however, feminist nurses "flexed their muscles" during the 1970s and early 1980s. Career-minded, influenced by a decade of social dissent, they now saw their professional and personal problems in a new light. The women's movement both explained the causes of their exploitation and offered solutions and alternatives. Feminist R.N.s — primarily younger, college-educated, employed in nursing's most elite fields — mobilized in a number of ways. They utilized trade journals, professional associations, educational institutions, and feminist nurse networks to spread their message. They engaged in consciousness-raising, allied themselves with like-minded women's groups, and supported constitutional guarantees of equal rights. Feminist nurses were not part of a monolithic front. Rather they represented various strands of the U.S. women's movement. They all, however, had learned to connect nursing to the larger questions of female inequality and sex discrimination.

Feminists nurses formed consciousness-raising groups and lobbied for the ERA. These, however, were not their only means of fighting inequality. Using a variety of strategies, nurses specifically fought sexism in their work places. Chapter 5 explores these tactics and their impact on the American health care system.

Endnotes

1. "1982 House of Delegates Action of the House," American Nurses Association Papers, Mugar Library, Boston University, 1-2, 7; "ANA Votes Federation," *AJN* 82 (August 1982): 1252-1253; "Continued Support for Equal Rights, Health Care Access Voted By House," *Convention News*, 30 June 1982, 1; "Emergency Resolution On Equal Rights for Women," 28 June 1982, American Nurses Association Papers, Mugar Library, Boston University; "Nurses Fill Lafayette Park," *Convention News*, 1 July 1982, 2; "Schafly to Hear from ANA," *Convention News*, 27 June 1982, 7.

2. David Chalmers, *And the Crooked Places Made Straight: The Struggle for Social Change in the 1960s* (Baltimore: The Johns Hopkins University Press, 1991), 162-163; Evans, *Personal Politics*, 15-21; Kessler-Harris, *Out to Work*, 313-314; May, *Homeward Bound*, 209-219.

3. Cott, "Feminist Theory and Feminist Movements," 58-60.

4. McLaughlin et al., *Changing Lives,* 48, 96, 120.

5. Cherlin, *Marriage, Divorce, Remarriage,* 22, 52-54; May, *Homeward Bound,* 6-8; McLaughlin et al., *Changing Lives,* 60, 127.

6. McLaughlin et al., *Changing Lives,* 170-174.

7. Evans, *Personal Politics,* 42-57, 64-76, 86-88, 99-101.

8. Cott, "What's in a Name?" 812-813; Evans, *Personal Politics,* 159-169, 193-194.

9. Linda M. Blum, *Between Feminism and Labor: The Significance of the Comparable Worth Movement* (Berkeley: University of California Press, 1991), 41; Cott, "What's in a Name?" 815; Evans, *Personal Politics,* 199-217, 231.

10. Blum, *Between Feminism and Labor,* 42-43; Mansbridge, *Why We Lost the ERA,* 105-107.

11. L.L. Dock, "Some Urgent Social Claims," *AJN* 7 (April 1907): 895.

12. Cott, *The Grounding of Modern Feminism,* 4-6.

13. For information on the ANA's opposition to the ERA during the 1950s and early 1960s see Nell V. Beeby, "Why the Equal Rights Amendment Was Opposed," *AJN* 60 (August 1960): 291; "Equal Rights Amendment," *AJN* 60 (August 1960): 1066; Janet Geister, The Equal Rights Amendment," 28 April 1954, American Nurses Association Papers, Mugar Library, Boston University, 152-158; Janet M. Geister and Ruth Addams, "The Equal Rights Amendment," *AJN* 54 (April 1954): 1061; "House Opposes Equal Rights Amendment," *Convention Journal,* 29 April 1954, 1; "Why the Equal Rights Amendment Was Opposed," *Nursing Outlook* 2 (June 1954): 291.

14. ANA, *Facts, 1968,* 20, 22.

15. ANA, *Facts, 1965,* 14; ANA, *Facts, 1968,* 16; ANA, *Facts, '72-'73,* 7, 16.

16. ANA, *Facts, 1969,* 7; ANA, *Facts, 86-87,* 10; Moses, "Nurses Today," 448; Moses and Roth, "Nursepower," 1746.

17. Moses and Roth, "Nursepower," 1747.

18. Nancy P. Greenleaf, "Labor Force Participation among Registered Nurses and Women in Comparable Occupations," *Nursing Research* 32 (September/October 1983): 309-310.

19. Chalmers, *And the Crooked Places Made Straight,* 174; Richard O. Easterlin, *Birth and Fortune: The Impact of Numbers on Personal Welfare* (New York: Basic Books, Inc, 1980), 113.

20. "A Plan for Fighting the Double Digits," *Time,* 18 April, 1977, 49; Harry Anderson, Erik P. Ipsen, Rich Thomas, "Good News on the Economy," *Newsweek,* 29 June 1981; "As Prices Keep Spiraling - How People Are Tightening Their Belts," *U.S. News & World Report,* 24 December 1973, 16; "Inflation Grows Worse," *Time,* 27 March 1978, 58; "No Crash of '79 Coming Up," *Time,* 2 October 1978, 54; "Why All The Talk Of Recession," *U.S. News & World Report,* 24 December 1973, 11.

21. Michael Goldfield, *The Decline of Organized Labor in the United States* (Chicago: The University of Chicago Press, 1987), 96-102.

22. Easterlin, *Birth and Fortune,* 128.

23. McLaughlin et al., *Changing Lives,* 115.

24. Subject #10, interview by author, tape recording, 23 June 1989, Mt. Carmel, Pennsylvania.

25. Subject #16, interview by author, tape recording, 13 July 1989, Harrisburg, Pennsylvania.

26. "California Hospitals See Many RNs Returning to Work," *AJN* 83 (January 1983): 34; Ross Mullner, Calvin S. Byrne, Suzanne F. Whitehead, "Hospital Nursing Vacancies," *AJN* 83 (April 1983): 547.

27. Kelly, "Goodbye, Appliance Nurse," 432.

28. Subject #3.

29. Judy Batson Smith, "Separation Anxiety: A Personal Experience," *AJN* 75 (June 1975): 972-973.

30. Subject #2.

31. Subject #17, interview by author, tape recording, 20 July 1989, Harrisburg, Pennsylvania.

32. Merton, "Relations Between Registered Nurses and Licensed Practical Nurses," 71.

33. Jacklyn Jones, "Letters," *AJN* 67 (April 1967): 748.

34. Janet Klein, "Letters to the Editor," *The Pennsylvania Nurse* 22 (May 1967): 2.

35. "Public Health Salaries Show Impact of Federal Controls," *AJN* 73 (November 1973): 11; Thelma M. Schorr, "Due for Attention," *AJN* 73 (November 1973): 1889.

36. Marjorie A. Godfrey, "Nurses' Salaries Today," *Nursing 77* 7(June 1977): 97.

37. Marjorie A. Godfrey, "The Dollars and Sense of Nurses' Salaries," *Nursing 79* 9(September 1979): 82.

38. Barbara Yacos, "Letters," *AJN* 72 (August 1972): 1389.

39. Marjorie A. Godfrey, "Nurses' Salaries Around the Country: Where You Can Earn the Most (And the Least?), *Nursing 74* 4(June 1974): 45.

40. Fourteen Authors, "Professional Care and Treatment," 79.

41. R.N. Michigan, "Letters," *AJN* 66 (February 1966): 264.

42. Leonard I. Stein, "The Doctor-Nurse Game," *AJN* 68 (January 1968): 103-104.

43. "Communication Discussed at AMA's Nursing Meeting," *AJN* 65 (August 1965): 22.

44. "M.D.s, R.N.s Trade Views on What Doctor Owes Nurse," *AJN* 66 (September 1966): 1909.

45. Ingeborg G. Mauksch, "Letters," *AJN* 66 (September 1966): 1952-1953.

46. Margaret L. Pluckhan, "A Problem Affecting the Delivery of Health Care," *Nursing Forum* 11, no. 3 (1972): 305-306.

47. Catherine Christiansen, "Letters," *AJN* 72 (May 1972): 886.

48. Subjects #3 and #4.

49. "Nursing Ethics, The Admirable Professional Standards Of Nurses: A Survey Report," *Nursing 74* 4 (September 1974): 37-38.

50. "Child Care Deductions," *AJN* 64 (January 1964): 18.

51. "ANA Asks Tax Benefits," *AJN* 69 (June 1969): 1148; "Child Care Deductions," 16.

52. Subject #18.

53. "Brookdale Nurses Find in Union There Is Strength," *1199 News*, October 1977, 10.

54. Mary Sather, "To Start a Child Care Center," *AJN* 72 (November 1972): 2062.

55. Subject # 9, interview by author, 22 June 1989, Carbondale, Pennsylvania.

56. Subject #8, interview by author, tape recording, 14 June 1989, Harrisburg, Pennsylvania.

57. Subject #10.

58. Barbara G. Schutt, "Confrontation," *AJN* 68 (May 1968): 997; Barbara G. Schutt, "Not By Bread Alone," *AJN* 69 (June 1969): 1205.

59. "Minorities' Sessions," *AJN* 71 (February 1971): 216; Barbara G. Schutt, "The Agony in Miami," *AJN* 70 (June 1970): 1241.

60. Barbara G. Schutt, "Power: Symbols and Substance," *AJN* 68 (October 1968): 2123.

61. Barbara G. Schutt, "What Do You Know About Hunger?" *AJN* 70 (January 1970): 65.

62. Julie Hoover, "Letters," *AJN* 70 (August 1970): 1658; Lynnae King, "Letters," *AJN* 70 (February 1970): 260; "Letters," *AJN* 70 (October 1970): 2098, 2100; "Letters," *AJN* 72 (April 1972): 652, 658; "Letters," *AJN* 72 (June 1972) 1065-1066.

63. By the early 1970s prominent nurses such as the ANA's executive director, Hildegard Peplau, and nursing educator, Ruth Freeman, had urged R.N.s to get involved. See "ANA's New Executive Director States Her Views," *AJN* 70 (January 1970): 84; Ruth B. Freeman, "Practice as Protest," *AJN* 71 (May 1971): 919-921.

64. "ANA on Rights Legislation," *AJN* 67 (November 1967): 2276; Irene Minor and Ethelrine Shaw, "ANA and Affirmative Action," *AJN* 73 (October 1973): 1738-1739; "Women's Civil Rights Group Joins New 'Mainstream,' " *AJN* 65 (March 1965): 48.

65. M. Phyllis Cummingham, Helene Richardson Sanders, Patricia Weatherly, "We Went to Mississippi," *AJN* 67 (April 1967): 801-804.

66. "Moratorium Day in Washington," *AJN* 70 (January 1970): 93; "Nurses March for Peace, Start National Group," *AJN* 70 (July 1970): 1403, 1406-1407; Subject #49, interview by author, 2 May 1991, Harrisburg, Pennsylvania; "Vietnam Veterans March in Brooklyn," *AJN* 71 (August 1971): 1500; "When the Veterans for Peace Marched on Washington, Nurses Were There," *AJN* 71 (June 1971): 1084.

67. Helen Donovan, "Can We Work with the Black Panthers?" *Nursing Outlook* 18 (May 1970): 34-35.

68. Subject #49.

69. Marion Moses, " 'Viva La Causa!' " *AJN* 73 (May 1973): 844-845.

70. Cunningham, Sanders, Weatherly, "Mississippi," 804.

71. Moses, " 'Viva La Causa!' " 844-845.

72. Cunningham, Sanders, Weatherly, "Mississippi," 804.

73. "Nurses March for Peace," 1407.

74. Schutt, "Power: Symbols and Substance," 2123.

75. Melosh, *"The Physician's Hand,"* 126-128; Reverby, *Ordered to Care*, 70, 110; Nancy Tomes, " 'Little World of Our Own,' " 469-472.

76. Gretchen Gerds, "The Status of Women Today and its Effect on Nursing," *AJN* 63 (November 1963): 70-73.

77. "Job Discrimination Facts Available in Pamphlets," *AJN* 67 (September 1967): 1818; "Women's Status Shows Rise in 1965," *AJN* 66 (July 1966): 1484.

78. For articles on sex discrimination see "U.S. Civil Service Commission to Hear Discrimination Appeals," *AJN* 71 (October 1971): 2000; "Women's Bureau Anniversary Has Women's Lib Aspects," *AJN* 70 (October 1970): 2053-2055; "Women's Economic Woes Told to Congressional Committee," *AJN* 70 (July 1970): 1412; "Women on University Faculties Paid Less than Men, OE Says," *AJN* 73 (August 1973): 1309; "Women Still Earn Less, Federal Study Shows," *AJN* 72 (April 1972): 770. For information on court decisions see "Sick Pay for Maternity Leave Mandated by Court," *AJN* 74 (June 1974): 1022, 1025; "Supreme Court Orders Equal Pay for Women," *AJN* 74 (August 1974): 1404; "Work Restrictiions for Pregnant Teachers Overruled," *AJN* 74 (April 1974): 604. For articles on abortion see "Gallup Poll Sows Majority Favor Legal Abortion, Birth Control Service for Teen-Agers," *AJN* 72 (November 1972): 1961; "OB/GYN Group Takes Stand on Abortion," *AJN* 72 (July 1972): 1311; "OB-GYN Group Takes Stand for Freer Abortion," *AJN* 70 (August 1970): 1754; "U.S. Courts Strike Down Restrictive Abortion Laws, British Nurses Ask Special Hospital Abortion Units," *AJN* 72 (May 1972): 867.

79. Subject #10.

80. Subjects #3, #4, #8, and #23.

81. Subjects #1 and #15.

82. Subject #1; Subject #12, interview by author, telephone, 28 June 1989; Subject #24, interview by author, 23 October 1989, Monroeville, Pennsylvania.

83. Teresa E. Christy, "Why I Am a Member of NOW," *AJN* 71 (February 1971): 265; Virginia Cleland, "Why I Am a Member of WEAL," *AJN* 71 (February 1971): 265; Ava Dilworth, "Why I Am Active in Women's Lib," *AJN* 71 (February 1971): 265; Nola J. Pender, "Why I Am for Equality for Women," *AJN* 71 (February 1971): 265.

84. Christy, "NOW," 265; Dilworth, "Women's Lib," 265; Pender, "Equality," 265.

85. Christy, "NOW," 265; Dilworth, "Women's Lib," 265; Pender, "Equality," 265.

86. Cleland, "WEAL," 265; Christy, "NOW," 265; Christy, "Voices From the Past," *AJN* 71 (February 1971): 288-290; Dilworth, "Women's Lib," 265; Ruth Greenberg Edelstein, "Equal Rights For Women: Perspectives," *AJN* 71 (February 1971): 294-298; Toby Golick, "The Amendment: Do Women Need It," *AJN* 71 (February 1971): 285-287; Pender, "Equality," 265.

87. Virginia Cleland, "Sex Discrimination: Nursing's Most Pervasive Problem," *AJN* 71 (August 1971): 1542.

88. Cleland, "Sex Discrimination," 1542-1547.

89. Nora Lacorte, "Letters," 71 (May 1971): 904.

90. Suzan Boyd, "Letters," *AJN* 71 (May 1971): 904.

91. Betty B. Parker, "Letters," *AJN* 71 (October 1971): 1908.

92. Wilma Scott Heide, "Nursing and Women's Liberation: A Parallel," *AJN* 73 (May 1973): 824-827.

93. Angela Barron McBride, "A Married Feminist," *AJN* 76 (May 1976): 754-757; Angela Barron McBride, "Can Family Life Survive," *AJN* 75 (October 1975): 1648-1653.

94. Donna Diers, Angela McBride, Ann Slavinsky, "Leadership: Problems and Possibilites in Nursing," *AJN* 72 (August 1972): 1445-1447.

95. Bonnie Bullough and Vern L. Bullough, "Sex Discrimination in Health Care," *Nursing Outlook* 23 (January 1975): 40-45; Thetis M. Group and Joan I. Roberts, "Exorcising The Ghosts Of The Crimea," *Nursing Outlook* 22 (June 1974): 368-372.

96. Audrey Berman, "Letters," *AJN* 73 (August 1973): 1321.

97. Mary Kay Burke, "Letters," *AJN* 73 (August 1973): 1320; Gloria Dubin, "Letters," *AJN* 74 (February 1974): 230; Prudence Gaines, "Letters," *AJN* 74 (February 1974): 230; E. Marjorie Sanford Garcia, "Letters," *AJN* 77 (March 1977): 398; Carolyn Innes and G. David Waldron, "Letters," *AJN* 74 (August 1974): 1974; Leslie H. Nicoll, "Letters," *AJN* 77 (January 1977): 40.

98. JoAnn Ashley, "About Power in Nursing," *Nursing Outlook* 21 (October 1973): 639-640.

99. Ashley, "Power in Nursing," 640.

100. Ashley, "Nursing and Early Feminism," 1466-1467.

101. Katherine B. Nuckolls, "Who Decides What The Nurse Can Do?" *Nursing Outlook* 22 (October 1974): 630.

102. Jeanne D. Fonseca, "On Being a Woman," *Nursing Outlook* 24 (April 1964): 227.

103. Gloria R. Smith, "Nursing Beyond the Crossroads," *Nursing Outlook* 28 (September 1980): 543.

104. Kathleen Boyle, "Power in Nursing: A Collaborative Approach," *Nursing Outlook* 32 (May/June 1984): 164-167; Tara Kamara, "Letters," *Nursing Outlook* 34 (January/February 1986): 8; Virginia M. Lange, "Letters," *AJN* 78 (June 1978): 994; Donna Moniz, "Putting Assertiveness Techniques Into Practice," *AJN* 78 (October 1978): 1713.

105. "ANA Convention '74," *AJN* 74 (July 1974): 1271; Subject #12.

106. "NLN Convention Report: Anaheim, California, April 24-27," *Nursing Outlook* 25 (June 1975): 379, 381.

107. "ANA Votes Federation," *AJN* 82 (August 1982): 1256; "Convention Special Report," *NLN News*, 6 May 1977, 8; "The Image of Nursing - How to Improve It," *NLN Convention News*, 26 April 1977, 9; Perspectives Committee, "Report," *1983 Business Book*, NLN Headquarters, New York, 38; Gloria R. Smith, "Models For The Clinical Practice Of Nursing in The 1980s: Alternatives And Issues," *1983 Business Book*, NLN Headquarters, New York, 38-42.

108. Nancy Fry Fasano, "Credit for consciousness raising," *Journal of Nursing Education* 16 (October 1977): 3-6; Phyllis Kritek and Laurie Glass, "Nursing: A Feminist Perspective," *Nursing Outlook* 26 (March 1978): 182-186; Barbara P. Madden, "Raising the Consciousness of Nursing Students," *Nursing Outlook* 23 (May 1975): 292-296; Janet A. Rodgers, "Struggling Out of the Feminine Pluperfect," *AJN* 75 (October 1975): 1655-1659.

109. Subject #26, interview by author, tape recording, 24 October 1989, Pittsburgh, Pennsylvania.

110. Subjects #1, #3, #4, and #15.

111. Bonnie Moore Randolph and Clydene Ross-Valliere, "Consciousness Raising," *AJN* 79 (May 1979): 922-923.

112. "ANA Joins Women's Lobby Day: Hits 'Sexism in Hospitals," *AJN* 81 (March 1981): 447; "ANA President Goes to the White House," *AJN* 76 (August 1976): 1220; "House Tackles Pay Equity Issue: Kennedy to Introduce Legislation," *AJN* 83 (January 1983): 7, 32; "Positive Response for Equality Hailed at Women's Conference," *AJN* 78 (January 1978): 9.

113. "ANA Honored by Women's Labor Group," *AJN* 79 (February 1979): 217; "Nurses Helped Put Ferraro Where She Is," *AJN* 84 (October 1984): 1305; "Women in the Federal Government: Status Static? Challlenges Issued," *AJN* 73 (February 1973): 208; "Women's Action Alliance Proclaims 'Agenda,' " *AJN* 75 (August 1975): 1270.

114. "California Nurses Issue Statement in Support Of Right to Abortion," *AJN* 78 (April 1978): 540; "Michigan Nurses Support Abortion Law Revision," *AJN* 71 (May 1971): 876.

115. "ANA Statement to Study State Legislation on Abortion," *Reports to House of Delegates, 1966-1968, Dallas, May 13-17, 1968*, American Nurses Association Papers, Mugar Library, Boston University, 62-63; "For Delegate Action," *AJN* 68 (April 1968): 788.

116. Joan Becka and Barbara Lograsso, "Letters," *AJN* 73 (May 1973): 795, 797; Sr. Beatrice Costagliola, "Letters," *AJN* 72 (March 1972): 450; Agnes Martins, "Letters," *AJN* 71 (January 1971): 48; Maureen E. Murnane, "Letters," *AJN* 70 (December 1970): 2548, 2550; Madeline Satwicz, "Letters," *AJN* 72 (February 1972): 242; Judith Unruh, "Letters," *AJN* 71 (May 1971): 908, 910; Claire Wankiewicz, "Letters," *AJN* 71 (March 1971): 474.

117. "League Sees Change," *AORN Journal* 34 (July 1981): 98; "Second Report From Las Vegas Convention," 5 May 1981, NLN Headquarters, New York.

118. Geister and Addams, "The Equal Rights Amendment," 710; "Why the Equal Rights Amendment Was Opposed," 291.

119. Geister, "The Equal Rights Amendment," 157; "The 1954 ANA Convention," *AJN* 54 (June 1954): 699-700.

120. Thelma M. Schorr, "A Good and Proper Stance," *AJN* 71 (July 1971): 1351.

121. Shirley Conn, "Letters," *AJN* 79 (September 1979): 1529; Cathy Remz, "Letters," *AJN* 80 (January 1980): 48; Fonda Sprehe, "Letters," *AJN* 79 (April 1979): 630.

122. "ANA Board Supports Equal Rights Bill," *AJN* 71 (July 1971): 1293.

123. "ANA Convention '76," *AJN* 76 (July 1976): 1126, 1129; "Nursing' Political Arm Names Director," *AJN* 74 (December 1974): 2147; Diane J. Powell, "The Struggles Outside Nursing's Body Politic," *Nursing Forum* 15, no. 4 (1976): 358.

124. "ANA Convention 1978," *Nursing Outlook* 78 (August 1978): 506; "ANA Convention '78: Honolulu June 9-14," *AJN* 78 (July 1978): 1233; "Future ANA Conventions to Be Only in ERA-Ratified States," *AJN* 78 (April 1978): 533.

125. "Florida ERA Forces Find Fresh Support in Final Campaign," *AJN* 82 (February 1982): 226; "Nurses Carry Their Banners for the ERA in Washington," *AJN* 78 (August 1978): 1287; "Nurses Rally for Ratification Campaign in Key States," *AJN* 82 (February 1982): 213; "Oklahoma RNs Staff Phone Banks to Seek New Support for ERA," *AJN* 82 (February 1982): 222.

126. "Illinois Nurses Shift 1979 Convention to Wisconsin," *AJN* 78 (October 1978): 1612.

127. Elsa Brown, "Letters," *Nursing Outlook* 29 (September 1981): 492; Penny A. McCarthy, "Old Vegas and Other Anachronisms," *Nursing Outlook* 29 (June 1981): 347; "NLN Convention - April 24-27, 1977" *AJN* 77 (July 1977): 1095; "NLN's Convention '77/Special Report," *NLN News* 25 (May-June 1977): 4, 7; "NLN Resolution Approved by the NLN Membership," 21 May 1975, NLN Headquarters, New York, 9; "38,000," *NLN News* 23 (June-July 1975): 1-2.

128. "Nurses Form Own NOW," *AJN* 75 (February 1975): 200; Subjects #3 and #12.

129. Members, Nurses NOW, "Letters," *AJN* 74 (March 1974): 423.

130. "Communication Gap," *Progress Notes* 11 (Fall 1977): 3, courtesy of Nurses NOW; "National Organization For Women, *Nurses NOW: Philosophy, Strategies, and Tactics,* Special Collections, Hillman Library, University of Pittsburgh, 1-3; "Nurses NOW Becomes a National Task Force," *Pennsylvania NOW* 2 (April 1974):5; Subject #3.

131. "ANA Convention '74," 1271; *Progress Notes* 11 (Fall 1977): 1-8; Subject #12.

132. Peggy Chinn, "What's In Our Name???" *Cassandra: Radical Feminist Nurses Newsjournal* 1 (November 1982): 3; Gretchen LaGodna, "Cassandra: A Report Of Beginnings," *Newsjournal* 1 (November 1982): 1-2.

133. "ANA Convention," *Newsjournal* 2 (January 1984): 3; Jeanne De Joseph, "ANA Convention," *Newsjournal* 2 (May 1984): 1, 4; Gretchen LaGodna, "Letters," *AJN* 83 (January 1983): 44.

134. "Contact Women," *Newsjournal* 3 (January 1985): 28; "Contact Women," *Newsjournal* 3 (May 1985): 29.

135. Chinn, "What's in Our Name???" 4; LaGodna, "Cassandra," 1-2; "Local Chapter News," *Progress Notes* 11 (Fall 1977): 7; Michele L. Ondeck, "Nurses Now," 11 June 1973, Special Collections, Hillman Library, University of Pittsburgh, 5; Subjects #1, #4, #5, and #24.

136. This observation is based on personal and telephone interviews with nine Nurses NOW members conducted by the author between June and October 1989.

137. Penny Bresnick and Adrienne Roy, "Buffalo Web Report," *Newsjournal* 2 (May 1984): 21; Sharon Deevey, "Cassandra in Cleveland: A Report Of Beginnings," *Newsjournal* 2 (January 1984): 12-13; Adrienne Roy, "Buffalo Web Report," *Newsjournal* 2 (January 1984): 13.

138. Subjects #1, #2, #3, and #26.

139. Subject #2.

140. Members, Nurses NOW, "Letters," 423; Subjects #2, #3, #4, #5, and #12.

141. Subjects #3, #4, #5, #12, and #24.

142. Madelon M. Amenta, "Temporary Help Agencies: Help Or Hindrance To Care?" *Progress Notes* 2 (Fall 1977): 2; Subjects #2, #5, #6, and #23.

143. Subject #3.

144. Subject #12.

145. "Business Agenda Background," *Newsjournal* 3 (May 1985): 6; Anne Montes, "Dear Cassie," *Newsjournal* 3 (January 1985): 4; "Re-Sources," *Newsjournal* 1 (January 1984): 17.

146. "Announcements," *Newsjournal* 3 (September 1985): 28; "Booklet Re-View," *Newsjournal* 2 (May 1984): 16; "More Reading From Emma," *Newsjournal* 3 (May 1985): 21; "Re-Sources," *Newsjournal* 2 (May 1984): 19.

147. Bresnick and Roy, "Buffalo Web Report," 20-21; "Web Reports," *Newsjournal* 3 (May 1985): 28.

148. Peggy Chinn and Charlene Wheeler, "Report of the Gathering," *Newsjournal* 1 (September 1983): 4; "Summer Reading?" *Newsjournal* 2 (May 1984): 25; "The 10th Michigan Womyn's Music Festival," *Newsjournal* 3 (May 1985): 14.

149. "Join Now," *Progress Notes* 11 (Fall 1977): 6; "New National Coordinator," *Progress Notes* 11 (Fall 1977): 1; Subjects #2 and #3.

150. "Business Agenda Background,"6.

151. Chinn and Wheeler, "Report of the Gathering," 4-5; Deevey, "Cassandra in Cleveland," 11.

152. "Reports Of The 1985 Cassandra Continental Gathering," *Newsjournal* 3 (September 1985): 5.

153. Cott, "Feminist Theory and Movements," 52-54.

154. "ERA Update," *Progress Notes* 11 (Fall 1977): 1.

155. Montes, "Dear Cassie," 4.

156. Billie Kahn, "Celebration of Defiance," *Newsjournal* 1 (April 1983): 7-8.

157. Schorr, "A Good and Proper Stance," 1351.

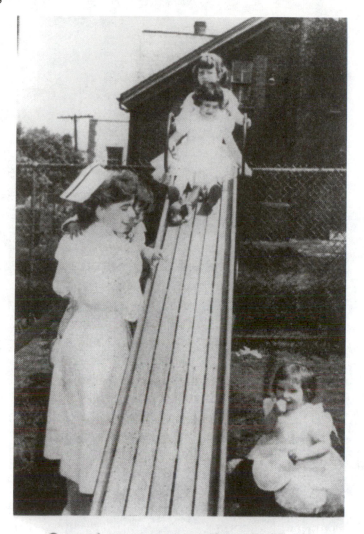

One of our nurse-mothers holds her
baby as she encourages another young-
ster to try out the playground equipment she and the other nurses helped
to purchase.

FIGURE 11

As a means of recruiting more nurses, many hospitals offered
on-site childcare in the 1950s and 1960s.

(Reprinted, by permission, from *Nursing Outlook*)

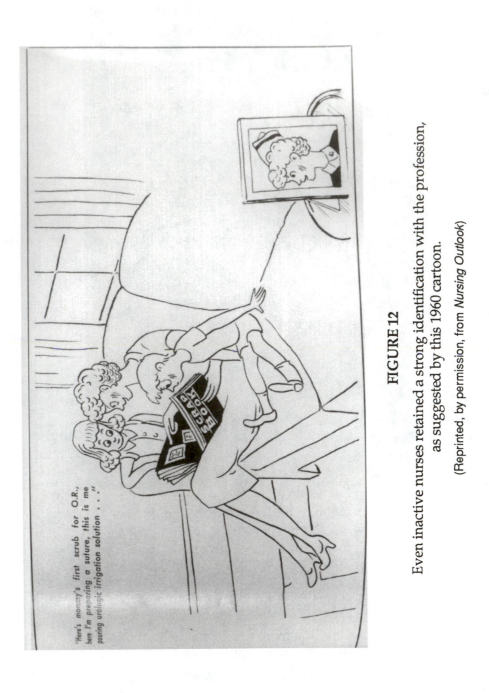

FIGURE 12

Even inactive nurses retained a strong identification with the profession, as suggested by this 1960 cartoon.

(Reprinted, by permission, from *Nursing Outlook*)

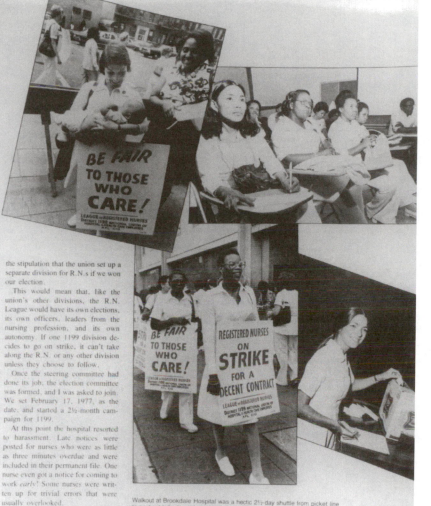

the stipulation that the union set up a separate division for R.N.s if we won our election.

This would mean that, like the union's other divisions, the R.N. League would have its own elections, its own officers, leaders from the nursing profession, and its own autonomy. If one 1199 division decides to go on strike, it can't take along the R.N. or any other division unless they choose to follow.

Once the steering committee had done its job, the election committee was formed, and I was asked to join. We set February 17, 1977, as the date, and started a 2½-month campaign for 1199.

At this point the hospital resorted to harassment. Late notices were posted for nurses who were as little as three minutes overdue and were included in their permanent file. One nurse even got a notice for coming to work *early!* Some nurses were written up for trivial errors that were usually overlooked.

The NYSNA suddenly entered the picture and flooded the hospital with campaign literature of its own. The NYSNA's previous efforts to organize Brookdale a few years ago had

Walkout at Brookdale Hospital was a hectic 2½-day shuttle from picket line to contract talks to, at last, a vote for settlement. The strike was punctuated by pleasanter moments relaxing with patients.

FIGURE 13

In the 1970s nurses increasingly used strikes
to resolve professional problems.

(Reprinted, by permission, from *RN*)

CHAPTER 5:

Work Place Feminism, 1970-1986

On January 23, 1986, 12,000 angry nurses struck 140 state-owned Pennsylvania health care facilities. For nine days the R.N.s picketed in subzero weather.[1] What led these women to leave patients and jobs for the picket line? Pennsylvania Nurses Association members fought for what they saw as a just cause — pay equity.[2] PNA unionists argued that the Commonwealth intentionally devalued their work because nurses were women. They demanded that the state upgrade job classifications and raise salaries.[3] As strike leader Ellen Willis explained, " 'People who take care of plants and cars [male maintenance workers] are paid more than nurses. Sex discrimination is occurring in the state and the state doesn't care.' "[4]

As had been true with pro-ERA demonstrations, nurses' strikes and calls for pay equity occurred with growing frequency during the 1970s and 1980s. Incensed over the working conditions discussed in Chapter 4, R.N.s were now increasingly likely to take action. More women joined collective bargaining units and negotiated contracts. Others reshaped the physicians' assistant movement in a way which afforded nurses more autonomy. Still others utilized the court system or left the profession in disgust.

Only a minority of nurses actually participated in these campaigns. Nor did all nurse-activists align themselves with the women's movement. But those most likely to consider themselves feminists — the nursing elite and college-educated baby boomers — were heavily involved in the movements discussed above. Their tactics and rhetoric showed an increasing awareness of sexism's impact upon nursing. Union members explained their activities from a feminist perspective. They negotiated over crucial women's issues such as daycare, maternity leave, and pay equity. Both liberal and radical feminists supported the nurse-practitioner movement as a way to free R.N.s and patients from medicine's domination. Litigation in the courts, under federal and state anti-discrimination laws, both acknowledged and attacked sexism. The early 1980s nursing shortage, fundamentally different from the post-World War II crunch, also had feminist overtones.

These strategies enabled R.N.s to raise salaries, improve working conditions and fringe benefits, and better juggle professional and family responsibilities. As nurses fought for their demands, they broke significantly with their past. They no longer acted like submissive and obedient girls. They behaved instead as women willing to confront injustice and eager to assume control of their profession. Work place feminism, however, could not completely resolve nurses' problems. The political and economic climate of the 1970s and 1980s created many obstacles. Each strategy had limitations and several carried risks for their users. This chapter explores these risks, as well as the issues, the tactics, and the actors involved in work place feminism.

Unionization

A small minority of nurses had joined CIO affiliates in the 1930s. During World War II the California Nurses Association also negotiated contracts for its members.[5] The ANA, afraid of competition from unions, implemented an Economic Security Program (ESP) and endorsed collective bargaining in 1946.[6] Organization proceeded very slowly. On the ESP's twentieth anniversary only four percent of nurses belonged to either an ANA or union-affiliated bargaining unit. Eight percent held membership in 1970.[7] Negotiating was also problematic. Because nurses lacked coverage under the National Labor Relations Act (NLRA), they could not force employers to come to the bargaining table. Furthermore, the ANA House of Delegates voluntarily relinquished one potential weapon — the strike — from 1946 to 1968.[8] Between 1960 and 1974 R.N.s nationwide staged a mere 103 work stoppages involving only three percent of practitioners.[9] The majority of these occurred after 1965.[10]

Nurses exhibited a new militance, however, in the 1970s and 1980s. Between 1972 and 1977 the percentage of unionized R.N.s grew from eight to thirteen percent.[11] The proportions increased to seventeen and twenty-two percent in 1980 and 1982, respectively.[12] While three-quarters belonged to state nursing associations (SNAs), the remainder joined national or local trade unions.[13]

Strikes occurred more frequently as well. Between 1970 and 1974 alone, nurses engaged in 232 work stoppages, a 58 percent increase over the previous five years.[14] In the latter 1970s the number of job actions virtually exploded. In 1976 Honolulu, Seattle, Chicago, and New York City experienced large-scale nurses' strikes. The New York walk-out disrupted forty-three hospitals and ten nursing homes. Between 1977 and 1979 Philadelphia, Pittsburgh, and Washington, D.C. witnessed lengthy hospital and public health strikes. By the early 1980s both the National Labor Relations Board (NLRB) and the courts reported themselves "flooded with cases involving nurses' organizations." Health care administrators expressed alarm over the "dramatic upswing" in R.N. militance.[15]

Job action rhetoric also changed. In the 1960s striking nurses emphasized patient care issues. They stated monetary demands indirectly. A retired SNA official recalled that when she began organizing nurses in 1967, "Everyone wanted money and benefits, but were afraid to say that, afraid it didn't sound proper."[16] In 1969, Cleveland R.N.s justified a seventeen week strike by linking patient care to salaries. In the words of one observer, the strikers

> stressed the responsibility of the nurse for high-quality work which in turn depends on satisfactory working conditions and personal job satisfaction. The appeal is to the nurses' spirit of craftsmanship. Hence, a nurses' strike is conceived not as a strike against patients, but as a way for nurses to gain benefits that will result in more and better care for patients.[17]

While patient care remained a concern, nurses stated their economic demands more straightforwardly in the 1970s and 1980s. Massachusetts and Minnesota strikers, for example, carried picket signs which read " 'Starve With Dignity, Be A Nurse,' " and " 'Nursing is my profession. It is not my hobby.' "[18] In 1986 PNA member, Sharon Demko, responded to public concern over patients by commenting, " 'Being nice doesn't pay bills and mortgages.' "[19]

Socal scientist have attributed this increase in nurses' organization and militance to the growth of public employee unionism and the passage of enabling legislation in the 1970s. In their analysis, a more favorable political climate and the examples of teachers, police officers, and firefighters encouraged R.N.s.[20] This interpretation, however, does not entirely explain their behavior. As John Burton and Terry Thomason argue, employee militance is not necessarily the *consequence* of legal legitimacy. Sometimes union organization actually *leads to* changes in labor laws.[21] Two well-publicized nursing incidents, the 1967 Brookville, Pennsylvania strike and the 1970 Hawaii job action are cases in point. No public employee collective bargaining law existed in either state at the time of the work stoppages. The NLRA would not include nurses until 1974. Brookville Hospital's strike also occurred one year before the ANA rescinded its no-strike pledge. In these two instances, then, R.N. militance predated both a favorable legal climate and the professional association's endorsement.[22] Furthermore, nurses did not immediately join unions after the passage of enabling legislation. According to Kathryn Grove, PNA executive director from 1968 to 1984, "There was no immediate flurry of organization after passage of Act 195 [Pennsylvania's 1970 public employee bargaining law]."[23] Nor did nurses rush to unionize after the passage of the 1974 Health Care Amendments to the NLRA. Instead, the largest numbers entered labor organizations between 1977-1982, the years of high inflation.[24]

Explanations which center on the changing legal climate also fail to account for demographic factors. Union membership grew most rapidly as baby boomers joined the ranks of nursing.[25] These younger women were the most ardent union supporters. A 1978 *RN* survey found, for example, that sixty-five percent of women under 35 years of age believed strikes were acceptable, compared to forty-seven percent of those over 35.[26] Four years later the magazine reported that sixty-one percent of nurses under 25, sixty-five percent of those aged 25-34, and forty-nine percent of R.N.s aged 35-44 supported unions. Only thirty-eight percent of those over the age of 44 agreed.[27] A 1985 poll likewise found that nurses under 45 years of age accepted unions and strikes more readily than older women.[28]

Baby boomers accepted unions because they perceived themselves as primary earners and long-term workers. Young R.N.s worried about inflation and realized they would likely be employed for a lifetime. Thus they saw union membership as an effective tool for improving working conditions. As a critical care nurse observed in 1978,

> When my grandmother was a nurse, back at the turn of the century it was understood that she would work for a year and then get married. Nursing would be something to fall back upon if her husband or children ever got sick. Nurses felt no need to strive for improved conditions, because they knew their jobs were only temporary.
>
> Today's nurses, married or not, can look forward to a career of 45 to 50 years. You and I, as nurses, may spend as many as 100,000 hours working...."[29]

Compare the above passage with the self-sacrificing tone of an older nurse's letter.

> When I graduated from nursing school in 1959, I was aware that the salary was low, the hours long, and the work load heavy. But I knew that when I went into nursing. These things haven't changed since then, except that inflation has made them more noticeable.

> The reason for my discontent is that doctors and *nurses* [italics mine] don't care any more.[30]

College graduates also saw collective bargaining as a means of acquiring salaries and benefits commensurate with their sense of professional status. A New York BSN described her union's 1977 strike in these terms.

> I was especially critical of the nurses' lack of a voice in their working lives.... We're told we're professionals but we're not treated as such. We're told it's unprofessional to unionize, yet the economic and working benefits that allow one to be a professional were going to unionized fellow employees.[31]

For baby boomers, unionization was also an effective feminist strategy. Establishing bargaining units and negotiating contracts became ways to challenge the health care patriarchy which discriminated against female workers. In New York City, Beth Israel Hospital's staff organized under 1199's auspices because "management looked upon us as little girls, not serious workers."[32] During 1978 thirty nurses, attending an 1199 conference, complained about sexism and called upon R.N.s to "overcome subservience."[33] Nurses from Connecticut and Texas who joined 1199 and SEIU in 1979, were also tired of employers who treated them like "children."[34]

Feminist groups, such as Nurses NOW, encouraged their members to organize. Nurses NOW's 1970s pamphlet, "Sexism In Nursing Is ...," effectively linked low salaries and unfair scheduling practices to gender stereotyping and exploitation.

SEXISM IN NURSING IS ...

working overtime because you are dedicated ... without pay,

working for peanuts, three shifts in one week, no extra pay for holidays or weekends, and working three weekends a month.[35]

Articles in the 1977 and 1978 newsletters likewise blamed poor working conditions on sexism and urged women to join SNA bargaining units.[36] In Pittsburgh, several Nurses NOW members struggled unsuccessfully to organize two local hospitals.[37] Another served as local unit president at a public health agency.[38]

For some nurses, unionization was itself a consciousness-raising experience. One PNA member had belonged to a local bargaining unit for several years when she walked into the newly renovated hospital lobby and suddenly realized, "Male wallpaper hangers made $10.00 an hour. Women in critical care made $4.30." As she linked this realization with her knowledge of the women's movement, she became a feminist.[39] Another local PNA officer, who had successfully negotiated several practice issues, came to see collective bargaining as a way to keep "male doctors from controlling women nurses."[40] A nursing instructor developed feminist consciousness during a 1980 negotiating session in which administrators' sexist attitudes led to a strike. She became aware that, "Most of the people on management's side of the table were male. The male-female authority-worker game had to be dealt with...."[41]

During the 1970s and 1980s nurses, like other unionists, negotiated higher salaries and better hours. But a feminist perspective also influenced collective bargaining. Nurses increasingly worked for contract provisions designed to benefit *women* workers. SNA and union members tackled problems stemming from the sexual division of labor within the family. According to a PNA organizer, nursing units negotiated "things which made [professional] practice and home life more manageable."[42] Contracts were thus likely to include clauses dealing with daycare, equity for part-time workers, and maternity leave and disability.

A note of caution must be interjected. Concern over female workers' special problems should not be automatically equated with feminist consciousness. As Nancy Gabin has argued, even sexist male UAW officials advocated maternity leave and on-site daycare in the 1930s and 1940s. Their efforts on women's behalf evolved from an interest in union growth and solidarity, not feminism.[43] Nancy Cott has likewise suggested that female consciousness, stemming from an acceptance of traditional sex roles, might also fuel demands for gender-specific benefits.[44] At least some nurses, however, saw these issues from a feminist perspective. Nurses NOW proposed childcare centers and maternity policies as ways of freeing R.N.s from the sexual division of labor.[45] PNA activists believed woman-centered benefits "empowered" working nurses.[46]

SNAs and unions thus negotiated parental leave, maternity disability pay, and pro-rated benefits for part-time employees.[47] At some worksites R.N.s fought harder for these issues than for salary increases. During an 1199 convention in 1979, one western Pennsylvania organizer reported that hospital staff nurses' major concerns revolved around maternity policies.[48] Throughout the 1970s R.N.s struck when employers refused to grant parental leave or equalize part-timers' benefits.[49] Nurses who worked at Rhode Island Womens and Infants Hospital joined 1199 precisely because their employer refused to reinstate new mothers. One activist explained her concerns:

> One nurse lost nine years seniority at Womens and Infants in 1969 after the
> birth of her sixth child. It [maternity leave] was the biggest thing in the ne-
> gotiations. It seemed as if they [management] were punishing us because
> we're women, punishing us for having a child.[50]

Nurse-unionists also dealt with women's issues away from the
bargaining table. Local units established their own daycare centers.[51]
Between 1974 and 1979 four of the largest organizers of nurses — the
ANA, SEIU, 1199, and AFSCME — passed convention resolutions which
supported parental leave and childcare policies.[52] The American Federation of Teachers adopted a childcare resolution in 1979, two years
after the union opened its membership to R.N.s.[53] Outside the convention hall, unions implemented these mandates in several ways.
AFSCME's national officers provided assistance to locals' daycare centers, lobbied for federal funding, and testified at Congressional hearings.[54] SEIU held women's conferences where delegates shared
strategies.[55]

Expanded Practice

While some nurses organized and negotiated, others advocated
new practice models. Many leaders, along with college-educated baby
boomers, placed great faith in the nurse-practitioner movement. As
nurse-practitioners, they argued, R.N.s could both gain control of their
profession and the respect of physicians. They also believed nurse-practitioners (NPs) were ideally suited to eradicate sexist practices which
exploited female patients. To facilitate expanded practice, supporters
also pushed for broader nurse practice acts, third-party reimbursement
for nurses, and hospital privileges for NPs.

The expanded practice movement was initially a response to developments within the medical profession. In the late 1960s physicians,
in short supply themselves, began training a new type of auxiliary
worker. These unlicensed physicians' assistants (PAs) worked directly
under M.D. supervision and relieved doctors of routine tasks.[56] Nursing leaders took a dim view of this trend. They argued that R.N.s, particularly those with graduate degrees and specialized knowledge, could
provide health care services without physician supervision. Educators
and administrators pointed out that nurses were excellently suited for
well-child and adult care, normal obstetric and gynecological cases,
management of chronic illnesses, and treatment of certain psychiatric
disorders. More efficient use of nurse-specialists, they maintained, was
a better means of allocating health care resources than training another
level of worker.[57]

By the early 1970s nursing leaders saw this expanded role as a professionalization strategy. They envisioned *nurse-practitioners* as autonomous professionals who worked outside the traditional hospital setting, away from meddling M.D.s. In a 1970 editorial, Edith Patton Lewis compared contemporary nurse-practitioners to Lillian Wald, who as a Progressive era public health nurse, "made house calls, prescribed and dispensed medications and treatments, delivered countless babies ... gave medical care and advice."[58] Leaders also believed that highly skilled NPs would finally win medicine's respect for nursing. Thelma Schorr argued, in 1972, that R.N.s functioning in expanded roles would shed their handmaiden image and become physicians' associates and partners.[59]

By mid-decade, however, expanded practice supporters also employed a feminist perspective. Advocates described the movement as a means of overturning male physician domination. Ingeborg Mauksch, in a 1975 article, saw NPs as the profession's liberators from M.D. sexism.

> The advent of woman's consciousness-raising combined with a newly acquired stance of assertiveness, enabled nurses to view and subsequently to understand their vassal-like condition. Gradually, along with women in general, nurses realized that the worth of their work had been deliberately undervalued. They also recognized they had served the wrong master....
>
> At last, there are signs of respect by nurses for nurses, and for nursing, the cement essential for building an autonomous, free, and respected group.
>
> The nurse practitioner seems to exemplify these changes. She recognizes the need for more egalitarianism in the practice setting.[60]

Two years later author Jacqueline Rose Hott expressed similar views.

> Although nurses would like to be thought of as competent, assertive, and accountable practitioners, the public image more closely resembles the turn-of-the-century stereotype of the nurse.... People still view the nurse as female nurturer, medicator, physician's assistant and maid.
>
> Some nurses [NPs], however, are assuming more independent, less timid roles.... Nurses' lib confronts physician chauvinism....
>
> We have an opportunity to change nursing' image from that of a quiet and submissive woman to that of a person seeking power....[61]

Supporters also believed expanded practice liberated female patients. During the 1970s feminist nurses increasingly criticized medicine for its patriarchal control of women's health care. Articles in the professional press described M.D.s as patronizing, cruel, and outright manipulative. In a trenchant 1975 article, Bonnie and Vern Bullough accused male physicians of deliberately "perpetuating misinformation" about female anatomy and psychology.[62] Feminists were particularly critical of the way in which medicine managed the birthing process. Ruth Lubic Watson, director of New York City's Maternity Center Association, observed that "women were disenchanted" with controlling and patronizing obstetricians and wanted "to be equipped to ensure their own health...."[63] Joan Mulligan, a student nurse-midwive, argued even more strongly that male physicians deliberately abused pregnant women.

> There truly seems to be something in the behavior of a pregnant woman about to birth a child which elicits a brutalizing and dehumanizing physician response. It is not too extreme to suggest that uterine envy is as viable a concept as penis envy.[64]

Feminists argued that nurse-practitioners and -midwives, rather than doctors, were best equipped to provide holistic, patient-centered health care. Three New York nursing educators, who had opened a private practice in the early 1970s, noted that the expanded role allowed them to be "directly accountable to the consumer" instead of "handmaidens to physicians."[65] Both liberal and radical feminists saw the nurse-practitioner movement as an important tool in the struggle for women's rights. The *AJN*, in 1980, characterized NPs and CNMs [certified nurse-midwives] as good health care providers for "women who don't want to be patronized, anesthetized, and placed in uncomfortable, abnormal positions."[66] Similarly Cassandra members viewed expanded practice as a way of combatting medicine's "partriarchal need to control all aspects of women's reproduction...." Nurse-midwives were professionals who could help women

> choose whomever they wanted to help them in the birth process in a place where they were comfortable and in control....[67]

Although NPs were never more than roughly one percent of all nurses, the movement did grow during the 1970s and 1980s. Between 1970 and 1984 the number of nurse-practitioners and -midwives rose from 2,000 to 22,000.[68] Most of this growth occurred after 1974 as nurses increasingly fought the use of physicians' assistants and discovered feminism.[69] The number of educational programs also grew from 131 to 199 between 1973 and 1980. Waiting lists, however, remained long.[70]

Nurse-practitioner schools attracted young, professionally-minded, college graduates. According to a 1977 survey, students' median age was thirty-five. Forty-five percent held professional association membership, twice the proportion of all registered nurses.[71] By 1980 eighty-three percent held college degrees.[72] These young women prized autonomy and collegiality. In 1975 a psychologist reported that students scored high on tests measuring achievement orientation and self-actualization.[73] NPs, responding to a 1980 poll, most frequently listed "independence" as the reason for choosing their specialties.[74] Loretta Ford, co-founder of the Pediatric Nurse Practitioner (PNP) program at the University of Colorado, observed that her students valued opportunities to make decisions about patient care and work collaboratively with physicians. [75]

Nurses who functioned in expanded roles practiced in a variety of ways. PNPs, for example, performed physical examinations and laboratory procedures, took patient histories, immunized children, instructed parents, and made home visits.[76] Mary Kohnke and her New York associates provided their clients with health teaching and home nursing. They also offered consulting services to local agencies.[77] By 1982 most nurse-practitioners worked in settings where a doctor was not physically present. Many NPs worked with low income patients.[78]

Nurse-practitioners, however, encountered several obstacles. State laws customarily forbid nurses from diagnosing and prescribing. Under these statutes, NPs and CNMs held a tenuous legal status.[79] Many physicians, fearing that nurse-practitioners might become competitors, opposed expanded roles. As Loretta Ford wryly commented in a 1972 speech, "Since the nurses accept it [the PNP program], the doctors will surely be against it."[80] State medical societies vigorously fought the speciality, lobbying state legislators for new restrictions on nurses. Hospital boards denied NPs access and refused to provide physician back-up.[81] Third-party insurance carriers balked at reimbursing nurses.[82] These obstacles particularly hurt women in private practice.

Nurse-practitioners interpreted these obstructions as patriarchal assaults on female independence. When the New York State Medical Society opposed a new and broader Nurse Practice Act in 1972, NPs wondered "if chauvinism is involved here."[83] In 1984 Illinois prosecuted CNM Kathy Regester for supposedly practicing medicine without a license. Two Cassandra members saw the arrest as an attempt to perpetuate female submission.

> the patriarchal state as represented by the Department of Registration is viewed as an agent of the oppressor. The nurse midwife is victimized by the rules under which the patriarchy works....

Kathy ws singled out for harassment because her economic success was threatening. Regester also exhibited "undesireable" female traits of intelligence, initiative, and independence....

By spelling out rigid rules the state demonstrated its control over every aspect of nurse midwives' practice. In the predominantly male profession of medicine, things are not spelled out. In its determination to control women who dare to be independent, the state demonstrates a double standard for monitoring professional practice.[84]

Feminist R.N.s advocated broader nurse practice acts as one means of fighting the health care patriarchy. They argued that amended laws legitimized expanded roles, facilitated autonomy, and made self-employment more feasible.[85] From the early 1970s through the mid-1980s professional associations lobbied for revisions. In 1973 alone thirty-nine SNAs tackled the issue of nurse practice acts.[86] After bitter feuds with state medical societies, they achieved a measure of success. By 1984 forty-three states had revised their nursing statutes. Twenty-six created a separate license for nurse-practitioners, seven allowed expanded roles for NPs and CNMs, and ten simply broadened their definition of nursing.[87]

By the late 1970s and early 1980s nursing associations also lobbied successfully for third-party reimbursement laws. Congress, in 1977, passed two landmark measures. Both the Inouye Bill and the Rural Health Clinic Services Act permitted Medicare and Medicaid to directly reimburse nurse-midwives.[88] In 1980 Maryland became the first state to require insurance companies to pay nurse-practitioners.[89] Others quickly followed suit. By 1984 seventeen states had passed third-party reimbursement laws.[90] In order to make headway, SNAs publicly de-emphasized the feminist perspective and stressed that the use of nurse-practitioners lowered costs. This appeal was very attractive to governments and a public concerned with a rising health care price tag.[91]

NPs fared less well on the issue of staff privileges. Institutional medical boards were reluctant to concede ground. Nurse-practitioners, who applied for hospital access, faced endless delays and red tape. Staff status often came with so many restrictions that the privilege was worthless.[92] Physicians also fought the issue through their professional associations. In 1983, for example, when the District of Columbia passed an admission privileges' ordinance, the local medical society countered by proposing more restrictive nurse licensing.[93] Even the Joint Commission on Accreditation of Hospitals' 1984 recommendation favoring staff privileges for nonphysicians proved problematic. The JCAH provided no sanctions for hospitals who refused to comply.[94]

Litigation

Because of both the barriers to professional practice and remaining economic inequities, nurses sometimes resorted to litigation. Initiating sex discrimination lawsuits had become a favorite liberal feminist strategy for women in male-dominated fields as early as the 1960s.[95] But nursing remained a feminized profession and courts interpreted the laws literally. Thus R.N.s had not joined other liberal feminists in utilizing this tactic.

During the 1970s nurse-educators, working in male-dominated academia, began to initiate litigation. Nursing professors sued in situations where they could charge employers with Equal Pay and Civil Rights Acts' violations. In 1970, for example, WEAL filed sex discrimination complaints against 300 colleges, citing inequities in salaries, promotions, fringe benefits, and workloads.[96] By mid-decade nursing professors at several prestigious schools had followed WEAL's lead.[97] The ANA, in 1973, charged several universities and the Teachers Insurance and Annuity Association with violations of Title VII. The nine college faculty who initiated the complaint accused TIAA of charging males and females the same premiums, but paying women roughly $200 less per month in retirement benefits.[98] These lawsuits affected relatively few R.N.s, since nurse-educators composed only three percent of all employed practitioners. Nevertheless this litigation exposed nursing's professional problems and set a precedent which other nurses could build upon.[99]

By the 1980s nurse-practitioners had also begun to use litigation. Their rationale was somewhat different from that of nursing educators. Because their problems stemmed from the barriers to practice discussed above, filing suit under the Equal Pay and Civil Rights Acts was not viable. Though feminist NPs interpreted physician interference as a form of patriarchal persecution, they had no clearcut means of proving sex discrimination. Nurse-practitioners, therefore, charged opponents with interfering with their right to earn a living. Two cases, *Sermchief v. Gonzales* and *Nurse-Midwifery Associates v. Hibbett*, illustrate how this strategy benefitted nurse-practitioners, -midwives, and their female patients.

The *Sermchief* case stemmed from doctors' opposition to a revised Missouri Nurse Practice Act. This law allowed nurse-practitioners to do procedures which had formerly been the preserve of medicine. The Act permitted them, for example, to perform pelvic exams and prescribe oral contraceptives. In 1980, under pressure from the state medical society, Missouri's Board of Healing Arts shut down four family planning clinics which employed NPs. Suzanne Solari and Janice Burgess, who worked at the Cape Girardeau clinic, filed suit in district court in 1982. Arguing both that they practiced legally and that no patients had filed complaints, Solari and Burgess charged the Board of Healing Arts with violating the Fifth and Fourteenth Amendments of the U.S. Constitution. After this Circuit Court ruled in the Board's favor, Solari and Burgess appealed. In late 1983 the Missouri Supreme Court ruled unanimously in favor of the women. The Court found their practice lawful, stating that NPs were fully qualified to asssess and diagnose.[100]

Solari and Burgess attracted widespread attention in the nursing press, which saw the case as a precedent. R.N.s from across the United States donated money for the second trial. Thirty nursing, public health, and family planning organizations filed friend-of-the-court briefs for the women.[101] The Supreme Court's decision was hailed as a victory in the war for nursing autonomy. In a public statement Carolyn Davis, executive director of the Missouri Nurses Association, praised the justices for recognizing nurses' "authority."[102] The *AJN's* Mary Mallison saw *Sermchief v. Gonzales* as welcome relief for "nurse-practitioners who've experienced psychological harassment from medical societies or boards."[103]

Nurse-Midwifery Associates v. Hibbett involved a similar issue. Controversy erupted in Hendersonville, Tennessee when obstetrician W. Darrell Martin and his nurse-midwife partners, Susan Sizemore and Victoria Henderson, applied for admission privileges at the local hospital. Hendersonville Hospital readily admitted Martin, but refused to extend access to the CNMs. The practice moved to Nashville, where again only Martin gained hospital privileges. After Sizemore and Henderson complained to the *AJN* in 1980, Nashville physicians harassed their partner. The State Volunteer Mutual Insurance Company cancelled his malpractice insurance. The distraught and discouraged physician left the state. In 1982 Sizemore, Henderson, and Martin sued the insurance company, five physicians, and three hospitals for restraint of trade. SVMIC settled a year later after the Federal Trade Commission ruled that the business had violated U.S. anti-trust laws.[104]

As had been true with *Sermchief v. Gonzalez*, coverage in the professional press was overwhelmingly supportive of Sizemore and Henderson. The case also took on a feminist perspective. The *AJN*, for example, accused the Nashville medical community of restricting pregnant women's "right to choose."[105] A nurse-midwifery student, writing for *Nursing Outlook,* believed the male physicians who opposed Sizemore and Henderson feared "loss of power ... over the child-bearing woman and the health care system itself."[106]

Pay Equity

Litigation did indeed help nurse-educators and -practitioners fighting for equitable salaries and benefits or the right to practice expanded roles. It did little, however, for the majority of R.N.s. Pay equity had much more potential for women who worked in jobs such as hospital general duty. Through unions and the court system, nurses worked on this issue during the 1970s and 1980s.

Pay equity, also called comparable worth, was developed by feminists as a strategy for raising wages in female-dominated occupations. Linda Blum defines the concept in this way.

> The different jobs that men and women perform can be compared in terms of requisite levels of skill, effort, responsibility, and working conditions; pay for women's jobs should be comparable to that for equivalently ranked male jobs.
>
> Its central premise - that women are as valuable as men and are equally entitled to a just "living wage," regardless of the value the market places on their work - contests the ideological underpinnings of the existing, unjust system.[107]

In one sense pay equity was the women's movement's response to criticisms that feminism benefitted only elite, white females in male-dominated jobs.[108]

Comparable worth appealed to nurses because it validated their credentials and work. It offered them a way to raise salaries and remain in nursing. R.N.s, for the most part, enjoyed their jobs and had no desire to enter male-dominated occupations. In her interviews with California nurses, Blum observed that all felt frustrated by nursing's low wages but none wanted to change fields.[109] JoAnn Ashley had made a similar observation in a 1980 article. Ashley believed women would not be happy if they left nursing for higher paying jobs. She warned that nurses would feel uncomfortable in male-dominated professions because "male professionals are possessive, jealous of any infringement of their rights and highly combative...." Instead she advised women to "value nursing and prioritize nurturing..."[110] By valuing women's work and compensating female workers accordingly, pay equity had the potential to do just that.

Nurses became familiar with comparable worth in several ways. During the late 1970s and early 1980s state governments, municipalities, and private agencies undertook pay equity studies. The evidence showed employers grossly underpaid R.N.s. AFSCME's Washington state survey, for example, found that nurses earned roughly the same as maintenance workers whose jobs received sixty-four percent fewer evaluation points.[111] During hearings before the California Commission on the Status of Women, a CNA official reported that R.N.s earned less than " 'stationary engineers, carpenters, electricians, and longshoreman.' "[112] EEOC investigations, reported in the professional press, also alerted nurses.[113] As R.N.s became aware of these findings, they mobilized.

Nurses found many ways to work for pay equity. Much of this activity took place through the professional associations. ANA officials testified before public agencies and served on the National Committee on Pay Equity's first Board of Directors.[114] The NLN and the ANA formulated comparable worth strategies at national conventions.[115] Both individual nurses and the professional associations became involved in pay equity lawsuits.

One of the earliest suits, *Lemons et al. v. City and County of Denver*, involved employees of Denver General Hospital and the Denver Visiting Nurse Service. In 1974, frustrated by years of unsuccessful negotiations, a dozen Denver nurses investigated the city's civil service rating system. What they found both amazed and enraged them. Fifty-eight, male-dominated jobs requiring less education, skill, and experience paid better than nursing. Hospital staff earned less than tire servicemen, tree trimmers, sign painters, and traffic signal mechanics. Top-level nursing directors received lower salaries than male supervisors with similar credentials and levels of responsibility. In response nine women filed a sex discrimination complaint with the EEOC in 1975. A year later they filed suit in federal district court.[116]

Nurses throughout the nation rallied to the aid of their Denver colleagues. The Colorado Nurses Association provided legal services and the ANA donated funds for an extensive job study. Both organizations ran news articles and solicited support from other SNAs. Financial contributions from R.N.s poured in.[117]

Despite this support, the 1978 trial proceedly badly for the nurses. Bonnie Bullough, who testified for the plaintiffs as an expert witness, was amazed by the blatant sexist behavior exhibited by some of the participants. During Bullough's testimony, Judge Fred Winner inter-

rupted to argue that the Declaration of Independence "doesn't say any-
thing about women." The city's lawyer insisted on addressing another
witness as "Mrs." despite the fact that the woman had earned a doctor-
ate in economics.[118] Judge Winner decided in favor of the defendants,
charging that comparable worth was not a valid concept under the
Equal Pay Act. Ruling for the plaintiffs, he stated, would "open
Pandora's box" and disrupt the economy.[119] The nurses promptly appealed and lost again in Federal Appellate Court. When the U.S. Supreme Court refused in 1980 to hear the case, *Lemons v. Denver* was
officially dead.[120]

In 1981 a more favorable court decision for female jail matrons,
County of Washington v. Gunther, and a supportive EEOC report, *Women,
Work, and Wages,* offered nurses a better legal environment.[121] Illinois
R.N.s won a comparable worth case on appeal in 1986. Wisconsin nurses
used a highly publicized trial, *Briggs v. the City of Madison,* to force their
employer to settle a pay equity grievance.[122] In 1987 hospital and prison
staff who worked for the Commonwealth of Pennsylvania received
$16 million dollars, "the largest pay equity award in the history of nurs-
ing."[123]

Comparable worth litigation, however, remained a difficult strategy to implement. Many courts continued to interpret statutes literally.
In the 1982 *Briggs* case, for example, the judge agreed that the city had
underpaid female public health nurses. Yet he maintained that Madison had not "intentionally discriminated" because it had "paid nurses
at the market rate."[124] In 1985 University of Georgia NPs lost their pay
equity suit because they could not convince the judge they performed
the same work as male physicians' assistants.[125]

Because of the difficulties involved with litigation, nurses also utilized collective bargaining to achieve pay equity. During the 1980s SNAs
and trade unions passed comparable worth resolutions, initiated job
evaluation studies, and negotiated pay equity contract clauses.[126] In
the words of an AFSCME unionist, collective bargaining was "the most
direct and expedient way to address pay disparity."[127] This approach
presented nurses with several advantages. As a lawyer observed in
1988, bargaining for comparable worth allowed women to avoid the
"intentional discrimination" test mandated by many courts.[128] PNA's
Economic and General Welfare program director believed negotiations
helped nurses build more solid legal cases.

> Even if you fail to achieve an appropriate remedy through negotiations, you
> could still seek redress through litigation and, in my opinion, the fact that

you made an effort to first seek redress through negotiations will be an additional factor in your favor should you go before a court.[129]

This strategy was indeed successful for state-employed PNA members. They negotiated a job study, conducted extensive bargaining sessions, and staged a highly visible nine-day strike before suing the Commonwealth in 1986.[130]

One of the earliest negotiated comparable worth victories occurred in San Jose, California. Here 1,350 hospital staff nurses walked off their jobs in 1982 after a year of unsuccessful contract talks. The key issue for the R.N.s was achieving parity with male pharmacists, medical technicians, and physical therapists. After a three month strike, the beleaguered hospitals signed a contract. Nurses did not win their initial demand, a thirty-seven percent raise over eighteen months. They did, however, receive a sizeable twenty-one percent increase over three years.[131]

Staff nurses employed by nearby Contra Costa County also gained a comparable worth contract in 1985. Encouraged by the San Jose victory, these CNA members formed a coalition with female clerical and social workers from AFSCME and SEIU. They then pressured the county supervisors to implement pay equity. Job studies had revealed that R.N.s earned roughly thirty-nine percent less than men in similar jobs. Still, the Comparable Worth Coalition fought a difficult and prolonged battle. The county argued both that job worth studies were not scientific and that it had no extra money for salaries. Management combatted all attempts to re-classify women workers. Ultimately, however, the nurses did receive pay equity adjustments in 1984 and 1986.[132]

During these job actions R.N.s stressed that discrimination, not lack of skill nor responsibility, created their low salaries. The Contra Costa County nurses, active unionists since the 1970s, "reframed their complaints in gender terms" after realizing the discrepancies between their salaries and those of male pharmacists and physicians' assistants.[133] In press releases and newspaper interviews other R.N.s also cited examples of glaring disparities between male and female workers. PNA members pointed out wage and retirement inequities between male prison guards and correction system's staff nurses.[134] Maxine Jenkins, CNA's labor representative, used a similar strategy in the San Jose negotiations. In an interview with the *AJN* she reported,

We'll be calling attention to the wages paid to craftsmen employed in expansion programs under way at San Jose hospitals. Carpenters and mechanics on these jobs are making $17 to $20 an hour. Construction workers are earning $15, nearly 50 percent more than most registered nurses.[135]

R.N.s also sought and received help from other feminists. *Ms.* editor, Gloria Steinem, joined San Jose strikers on the picket line.[136] Both the National Women's Political Caucus and NOW sent letters of support to the Contra Costa County nurses.[137]

A New Nursing Shortage

San Jose, Contra Costa, and Pennsylvania R.N.s struck or sued because they wanted to improve nurses' salaries. For other dissatisfied women, negotiations and litigation were not viable strategies. These nurses left the profession.

By the mid-1980s the shortage, which had lessened somewhat earlier in the decade, returned. In 1984 the AHA reported that one in three hospitals had difficulty hiring and retaining nurses. Sixteen percent of the respondents experienced a moderate to serious problem. Almost all expected the shortage to worsen.[138] Between 1985 and 1986 the nationwide hospital vacancy rate for nurses doubled, rising from 6.5 to 13.6 percent.[139] Health care recruiters, meeting in Kansas City during 1986, predicted, "We'll be in a pickle by 1990."[140] Nurses with graduate degrees were particularly scarce.[141] In 1984 the U.S. had three times as many jobs as MSNs to fill them.[142] Hospitals offered extra fringe benefits to attract desperately needed critical care specialists.[143] Drops in nursing school enrollments after 1983 heightened anxiety about the R.N. shortage.[144]

This new shortage differed fundamentally from the deficit of the postwar era discussed in Chapter 2. In the 1950s and 1960s American health care's tremendous expansion had created demand for massive numbers of nurses. In the mid-1980s, however, vacancies occurred as dissatisfied women left the profession. After decades of fighting unsatisfactory wages and working conditions, R.N.s finally "voted with their feet." The most disgruntled nurses were those with the highest educational levels. One survey found, for example, that fifty-three percent of R.N.s with doctorates would not again choose nursing as a career.[145]

Well-educated members of the nursing elite found their economic rewards lacking, compared to those of professionals in male-dominated fields. During the 1980s R.N.s seemed particularly disgusted with wage compression. While some male professionals could expect their incomes to grow three hundred percent during their working lives, nurses' salaries increased only twenty-seven percent.[146] One University of Texas study found that twenty year veterans earned only $2,000 more annually than new graduates.[147] As nursing historians Philip and Beatrice

Kalisch observed, "There is no incentive to remain a working nurse."[148]

Nurses also remained dissatsified with working conditions. Collective bargaining, expanded roles, and litigation had not alleviated all problems in this area. Professionally-minded R.N.s complained about employers who expected them to perform non-nursing functions. In a 1982 *AJN* survey, ninety percent of respondents had to regularly work at housekeeping chores such as stacking towels and moving beds. Ninety-two percent said these duties lowered their job satisfaction.[149] Younger women with children were tired of working rotating shifts and weekends. As a nursing director admitted in 1986, "We don't have any problems filling positions in radiology or outpatient surgery, where the nurses work five days a week, 9-5."[150] Doctor-nurse conflict also contributed to the exodus. Both the University of Texas and the Medical Association of Alabama published studies which cited physicians as a primary reason for R.N. dissatisfaction.[151]

Certainly not all exiting nurses were feminists. There is no question, however, that the women's movement contributed to the way in which R.N.s defined their professional problems. Feminism had encouraged nurses to raise their sights and to expect fair treatment. As a University of Texas educator wrote,

> The shortage of nurses is an effective demonstration of positive changes in the status of women.
>
> Nurses are no longer willing to accept the subservient roles imposed upon them by society and the health care system.[152]

Lucie Young Kelly also saw nurses' discontent as a result of both women's heightened expectations and awareness of sex-role stereotyping. In a 1984 article about nurses with doctorates she noted,

> About 50 percent [of surveyed Ph.D.s] reported that their career preference today would be medicine, business or law ... just the fields, once not as accessible to women.... In those fields, they say, there's more money and status....[153]

Nowhere was feminism's impact more noticeable than on the career choices of women enrolling in college during the 1980s. This generation had grown up with the women's movement, saw themselves as lifetime workers, and believed they could succeed in any occupation they chose. They entered formerly male fields — business, medicine, and law. Fewer opted for the typically female professions of nursing and teaching.[154]

The Limitations of Work Place Feminism

Throughout the 1970s and 1980s nurses developed several feminist strategies to deal with professional issues. But unionization, expanded roles, litigation, pay equity, and withdrawal could not completely resolve work place problems. The political and economic climate, particularly in the 1980s, created many obstacles for nurse-activists. Other dilemmas also limited the usefulness of these tactics.

Collective bargaining had one obvious limitation. Despite increased union activity, three-quarters of nurses were still unorganized by the mid-1980s. Other problems also restricted labor's effectiveness. Inclusion within the NLRA did not end difficulties over union recognition. After 1974 employers argued that registered nurses were supervisors and thus ineligible for collective bargaining.[155] Nurse-activists complained of vicious, well-financed, union busting campaigns.[156] Such tactics obviously hampered efforts to organize. Health care cost containment programs, initiated during the late 1970s and early 1980s, limited contract settlements.[157]

Nurse-practitioners and -midwives also faced many obstacles. Wages and working conditions did not live up to women's expectations. In 1985 two *RN* editors reported that "NP salaries are far from special."[158] Nurse-practitioners faced considerable stress in the form of heavy workloads, patient demands, and conflicts with both physicians and other R.N.s.[159] NPs and CNMs had frequent run-ins with insurance companies, even in states with favorable reimbursement laws. Procedural problems and complex regulations made it difficult for nonphysicians to actually collect their fees. Federal and state agencies were no more responsive than private carriers. One year after passage of the Rural Health Clinic Services Act, only eight percent of eligible providers received federal funds.[160]

As states amended nurse practice acts and insurance laws, physician challenges accelerated. Bonnie Bullough reported that NPs and CNMs faced seventeen legal actions between 1974 and 1983. In eighty-three percent of these cases, state medical societies opposed nurses' right to practice.[161] The New Jersey and Kansas Medical Societies, in 1978 and 1981, charged nurse-practitioners with the illegal practice of medicine.[162] A year after Oregon NPs won direct reimbursement and the right to prescribe, the state medical association sponsored a bill designed to sharply curtail these privileges.[163] In 1981 and 1982 Louisiana and Texas physicians challenged their respective Board of Nursings' rights to regulate expanded practice.[164] For nurse-practitioners, the struggle for autonomy seemed never-ending.

The Equal Pay and Civil Rights Acts proved as difficult to implement as nurse-practitioner legislation. Because of foot-dragging and legal manuevering, many plaintiffs waited years to have their cases heard. When nurses got their "day in court" the results were often disheartening. In 1979, for example, a judge dismissed *Spaulding, et al. v. the University of Washington*. He claimed the nursing faculty failed to prove discrimination.[165] Successful litigation set plaintiffs up for potential retaliation. As Virginia Cleland observed, "Lawsuits always carry a career risk."[166]

Women encountered additional problems as they worked for pay equity. Although government-employed nurses made gains, little spillover occurred in the private sector.[167] Employers resisted using job evaluation studies to determine salaries. The job studies themselves carried a potential risk. As Linda Blum cautioned,

> the success of the movement hinges on its handling of technical measurement issues.... There is an ever-present threat that managerial control of the job evaluation methodology will compromise the interests of low-paid women while at the same time obscuring this fact.[168]

The ultimate tactic, leaving the profession, was perhaps the least adequate of all. While women found better wages in other jobs, many missed the satisfaction they'd felt as nurses. One, who left the profession in 1981 confessed, "That [quitting] made me sad because I love my work."[169] A former nurse turned business owner explained, "I opened my business for personal reasons [dislike of rotating shifts, weekend and holiday work]. I had no problem with nursing per se."[170]

While feminist nurses struggled to reform their work places, they encountered rejection in the larger society. The women's movement, concerned with breaking down barriers in male-dominated professions, sometimes rejected nurses. The conservative backlash of the 1980s also made it more difficult to implement feminist agendas. Media depictions of "women's libbers" as strident, unfeminine man-haters alienated R.N.s who might otherwise have been sympathetic. Furthermore many nurses, particularly older women educated and employed in hospitals, rejected the women's movement's tenets. Chapter 6 explores these obstacles to feminism.

Endnotes

1. "Nurses Back On Job At State Facilities," *The Daily American (Somerset, Pennsylvania),* 1 February 1986, 8; Pat Purcell, "Strike Talks Continuing," *Pottsville (Pennsylvania) Republican,* 30 January 1986, 17; "State Nurses Take To Picket Lines," *The Daily American,* 23 January 1986, 2.

2. Supporters of pay equity, also known as comparable worth, believe society devalues women's work. They argue that traditional women's jobs are as valuable as men's and that women workers are equally entitled to a fair, living wage. See Blum, *Between Feminism and Labor,* 2.

3. "State Nurses Take To Picket Lines," 2; Zakaria Tabassum, "State Seeks Court Order To Force Nurses To Work," *Pottsville Republican,* 23 January 1986, 6.

4. Robert Curran, "Strike Impending At 3 Regional State Hospitals," *The Tribune (Scranton, Pennsylvania),* 19 January 1986, B1.

5. Reverby, *Ordered to Care,* 197; Wagner, "Proletarianization of Nursing," 283-284, 288.

6. "American Nurses' Association activities," *AJN* 46 (November 1946): 728-729.

7. Marjorie E. Godfrey, "Nurses Salaries," *Nursing 74* 4 (June 1974): 57; Joel Seidman, "Nurses And Collective Bargaining," *Industrial and Labor Relations Review* 23 (April 1970): 343.

8. For information on the ANA's no-strike pledge see "American Nurses' Association activities," 728-729; "For Delegate Approval," *AJN* 68 (April 1968): 789; "Resolution Re ANA ES Policies," *Convention Journal,* 17 May 1968, 2; "Support For SNA's In Economic Action," *Convention Journal,* 17 May 1968, 1-2. For a discussion on nurses' NLRA exemption see "ANA Launches Drive to Organize Nurses for Collective Action on Quality Care," *AJN* 74 (January 1974): 7; "ANA Suggests Cotton Bill Not Wisest Solution," *AJN* 67 (September 1967): 935; "ANA Testifies on Taft-Hartley Exemption," *AJN* 73 (October 1973): 1667; "Asks Congress to Repeal Hospital Exemption," *AJN* 72 (February 1972): 195; "New Climate for Nurses in Nation's Capital," *AJN* 67 (May 1967): 935; William C. Scott, Elizabeth K. Porter, Donald W. Smith, "The Long Shadow," *AJN* 66 (March 1966): 543; "Taft-Hartley Exemption May End," *AJN* 72 (October 1972): 1772.

9. Michael H. Miller and Lee Dodson, "Work Stoppage Among Nurses," *Journal of Nursing Administration* 6 (December 1976): 43.

10. Department of Labor, *Impact of the 1974 Health Care Amendments to the NLRA on Collective Bargaining in the Health Care Industry* (Washington, D.C., 1979), 320.

11. Roger Feldman and Richard Scheffler, "The Union Impact On Hospital Wages And Fringe Benefits," *Industrial and Labor Relations Review* 35 (January 1982): 203; Edward C. Kokklenberg and Donna R. Sockell, "Union Membership in the United States, 1973-1981," *Industrial and Labor Relations Review* 38 (July 1985): 505.

12. Leon Fink and Brian Greenberg, *Upheaval in the Quiet Zone: A History of Hospital Workers Union, Local 1199* (Urbana: University of Illinois Press, 1989), 171;

Kokklenberg and Sockell, "Union Membership," 505; Anthony Lee, "A Wary New Welcome For Unions," *RN* 45 (November 1982): 36; "Six surprising facts about unions and nursing," *RN* 43 (July 1981): 43.

13. Fink and Greenberg, *Upheaval in the Quiet Zone*, 171; Lee, "A Wary New Welcome," 36; "Organized RNs Earn 17% More Than Unorganized RNs," *1199 News* 12 (August 1975): 26; "Six surprising facts," 43.

14. *Impact of the 1974 Amendments*, 320.

15. Gail Bentivegna, "Labor Relations: Union Activity Increases Among Professionals," *Hospitals* 53 (April 1, 1979): 134-136; Clifton L. Elliot, "Hospitals must face heavy unionization drives in '80s - part 1," *Hospitals* 55 (June 16, 1981): 55; *Impact of the Health Care Amendments*, 320; Jerome A. Koncel, "Hospital Labor Relations Struggles Through Its Own Revolution," *Hospitals* 51 (April 1, 1977): 70-71; Norman Metzger, "Hospital Labor Scene Marked By Union Issues," *Hospitals* 54 (April 1, 1980): 105-106.

16. Subject #7, interview by author, 14 June 1989, Camp Hill, Pennsylvania.

17. Norma K. Grand, "Nightingalism, Employeeism, and Professional Collectivism," *Nursing Forum* 10, no. 3 (1971): 294.

18. "Staffing, Salaries, and Safety Issues Prompt Strike at Lynn, Mass," *AJN* 83 (August 1983): 1120; "Twin Cities RNs Win On Issue Of 'Unfair' Layoffs," *AJN* 84 (August 1984): 1049.

19. Pat Purcell, "Nurses Strike at Ashland, Coaldale," *Pottsville Republican*, 22 January 1986, 6.

20. John Thomas Delaney, "Union Success in Hospital Representation Elections," *Industrial Relations* 20 (Spring 1981): 150-151; Kokklenberg and Sockell, "Union Membership," 501-502; David Lewin and Shirley B. Goldenberg, "Public Sector Unionism in the U.S. and Canada," *Industrial Relations* 19 (Fall 1980): 239-240; *Impact of the Health Care Amendments*, 33-41; Helene S. Tanimoto and Gail F. Inaba, "State employee bargaining: policy and organization," *Monthly Labor Review* 108 (April 1985): 51-52.

21. John F. Burton, Jr. and Terry Thomason, "The Extent of Collective Bargaining in the Public Sector," in *Public Sector Bargaining*, eds. Benjamin Aaron, Joyce M. Najita, and James L. Stern (Washington, D.C.: The Bureau of National Affairs, Inc, 1988), 18-19, 27.

22. Kathryn J. Grove, interview by Alice M. Hoffman, *Kathryn J. Grove, Executive Director, 1968-1984, PNA Oral History Interviews, 1984-85*, Dorothy M. Novello Memorial Library, The Pennsylvania Nurses Association, Harrisburg, Pennsylvania, III-24-III-25; Paul D. Staudohar, "The Emergence Of Hawaii's Public Employment Law," in *Public Sector Labor Relations: Analysis and Readings*, eds. David Lewin, Peter Feuille, and Thomas Kochan (New York: Thomas Horton and Daughters, 1977), 64-67.

23. Grove interview, III-41.

24. Feldman and Scheffler, "The Union Impact," 203; Fink and Greenberg, *Upheaval*

in the Quiet Zone, 171; Kokklenberg and Sockell, "Union Membership," 505; Lee, "A Wary New Welcome," 36; "Six surprising facts," 43.

25. ANA, *Facts, 86-87,* 10; Moses, "Nurses Today," 448; Moses and Roth, "Nursepower," 1746.

26. Lynn Donovan, "Is Nursing Ripe For A Union Explosion?" *RN* 41 (May 1978): 63.

27. Lee, "A Wary New Welcome," 38.

28. Debra Brewin-Wilson, "How wide is the generation gap in nursing?" *RN* 48 (September 1985): 28.

29. Maria Telesco, "Let's say 'yes' to unions!" *RN* 41 (October 1978): 34.

30. Constance S. Preble, "Letters," *Nursing 75* 5 (July 1975): 6.

31. Debra Wynne, "A Union Contract Was The Only Language Our Hospital Would Understand," *RN* 41 (May 1978): 66.

32. "Beth Israel's 675 Nurses Join 1199's RN Divison," *1199 News* 13 (September 1978): 6.

33. "RN Weekend Institute," *1199 News* 13 (July 1978): 30-31.

34. "Another Big Win In Connecticut," *1199 News* 14 (March 1979): 5; "The Dawn of a New Day," *Service Employee* 38 (September 1979): 10.

35. Nurses NOW, "Sexism In Nursing Is...," Special Collections, Hillman Library, University of Pittsburgh, 2.

36. Anne Butz, "Collective Bargaining," *Progress Notes* 2 (1977): 3; "From the National Coordinator," *Progress Notes* 3 (Winter 1978): 2-3.

37. Subjects #3, #5, #12, #24.

38. Subject #6.

39. Subject #10.

40. Subject #20, interview by author, telephone, 28 August, 1989.

41. Ruth Korn, "Nurses United! One Staff's Decision to Strike," *AJN* (December 1980): 2221.

42. Subject #8.

43. Nancy F. Gabin, *Feminism in the Labor Movement: Women And The United Auto Workers, 1935-1975* (Ithaca: Cornell University Press, 1990), 21, 76, 80-81.

44. Cott, "What's in a Name?" 827.

45. Nurses NOW, "Philosophy, Strategies, And Tactics," 10.

46. Subjects #8 and #20.

47. For information on SNA and union negotiated parental leave see "Around The Locals," *Service Employee* 34 (April 1975): 8; "Collective Bargaining Builds Momentum/Strength in Pennsylvania," *The Pennsylvania Nurse* 36 (October 1981): 10; "New SNA Contracts," *AJN* 83, 84 (October 1983-July 1984); "Professional-

ism Through An 1199 Contract," *1199 News* 14 (April 1979): 27; "Providence Nurses Win Voice in Policy Making," *AJN* 76 (February 1976): 181; Subject #16; "Wage And Benefit Gains in Elmwood Manor Pact," *1199 News* 16 (March 1981): 10. For a discussion of maternity disability pay in contracts see "Brookdale RN Wins Maternity Disability Pay," *1199 News* 15 (February 1980): 22; "New SNA Contracts," *AJN* 84 (March 1984): 378; "Ruling Goes in PNA's Favor at Polyclinic," *The Pennsylvania Nurse* 39 (January 1984): 5. For part-time workers' benefits see "Around the Locals," *Service Employee* 39 (May 1980): 10; "Carrier Pact Breaks New Ground for Jersey RNs," *1199 News* 17 (February 1982): 20; "Community RNs Gain Contract Imrovements," *1199 News* 13 (February 1975): 9; "Easton Hospital Settles," *The Pennsylvania Nurse* 40 (June 1985): 8; "First RN Contract At Jamaica Averts Strike," *1199 News* 12 (October 1977): 14; "New SNA Contracts," *AJN* 84, 85 (June 1984-November 1985); "Providence Hospital RNs Ratify Contract," *AJN* 80 (July 1980): 1244; "R.I. Nurses' First 1199 Pact Brings $70 Hike," *1199 News* 12 (January 1977): 10; Subject #19, interview by author, 28 August 1989, Philadelphia, Pennsylvania; "$24 raises for 250 at Miners Hospital," *1199 News* 10 (June 1975): 20.

48. "District Organizing Reports," *Minutes, Fourth Convention Of the National Union of Hospital and Health Care Employees, December 5, 1979,* New York State School of Industrial and Labor Relations, Martin P. Catherwood Library, Labor-Management Documentation Center, Cornell University.

49. "DC Nurses Strike Capital's Largest Private Hospital," *AJN* 78 (July 1978): 1146; "Nurses Make Hospital Cough Up Better Pact," *Service Employee* 42 (November 1982): 8; "Respect Was The Issue in Holden Strike Victory," *1199 News* 20 (March 1985): 22; "230 Ohio RNs Vote 1199," *1199 News* 16 (January 1981): 8; "Victory in Rhode Island," *1199 News* 15 (February 1980): 3.

50. "Rhode Island RN says: 'Management penalized us for pregnancies until we got our union contract,' " *1199 News* 12 (February 1975): 19.

51. "A First in Day Care For 1199er's Kids," *1199 News* 17 (August-September 1982): 15; "Child Care Is A Burning Need," *Service Employee* 39 (April 1980): 8; "On the Economic Scene," *AJN* 81 (July 1981): 1264; "Pushing Women's Rights in the Reagan Era," *1199 News* 21 (February 1986): 13.

52. "Bills Would Prohibit Pregnancy Inequities," *AJN* 77 (May 1977): 778; "Childcare," *Fourth Convention Of the National Union of Hospital and Health Care Employees, December 5, 1979,* New York State School of Industrial and Labor Relations, Martin P. Catherwood Library, Labor-Management Documentation Center, Cornell University; "Coalition Asks Sick Pay Equity," *Service Employee* 36 (April 1977): 5; "Resolution 62," *AFSCME Convention Proceedings, 20th International Convention,* Honolulu, Hawaii, 10-14 June, 1974, New York State School of Industrial and Labor Relations, Martin P. Catherwood Library, Labor-Management Documentation Center, Cornell University.

53. "Action on Resolutions," *Convention Reports, 1979, American Federation of Teachers, AFL-CIO, Sixty-Third Annual Convention,* San Francisco, California, 2-6 July 1979, New York State School of Industrial and Labor Relations, Martin P. Catherwood Library, Labor-Management Documentation Center, Cornell University, 16, 23; "Committee Reports," *Convention Reports, 1979, American Federation of Teachers,* 1, 5.

54. "Department of Legislation and Political Education," *Proceedings of the 22nd International Convention, Miami Beach, Florida, 14-18 June 1976, American Federation of State, County, and Municipal Employees, AFL-CIO,* New York State School of Industrial and Labor Relations, Martin P. Catherwood Library, Labor-Management Documentation Center, 346; "Report of the Community Non Profit Committee," *Proceedings of the 22nd International Convention,* 166.

55. "Women's Issues Focus of SEIU Conference," *Service Employee* 40 (March 1981): 2.

56. Kathleen G. Andreoli and Eugene A. Stead, Jr., "Training Physicians' Assistants at Duke," *AJN* 67 (July 1967): 1442-1443; Thelma Ingles, "A New Health Worker," *AJN* 68 (May 1968): 1059; Henry Silver and Loretta Ford, "The Pediatric Nurse Practitioner at Colorado," *AJN* 67 (July 1967): 1443-1444; Joseph Stokes, III, "More Physicians, More Highly Trained Nurses, or a New Health Worker?" *AJN* 67 (July 1967): 1441-1442.

57. Ava S. Dilworth, "Joint Preparation for Clinical Nurse Specialists," *Nursing Outlook* 18 (September 1970): 22-25; Edith P. Lewis, "The Invisible Nurse," *Nursing Outlook* 19 (March 1971): 157; Dorothy Mereness, "Recent Trends in Expanding Roles of the Nurse," *Nursing Outlook* 18 (May 1970): 32.

58. Edith P. Lewis, "The Nurse Practitioner," *Nursing Outlook* 18 (May 1970): 29.

59. Thelma M. Schorr, "An Important Distinction," *AJN* 72 (September 1972): 1581.

60. Ingeborg G. Mauksch, "Pro," *AJN* 75 (October 1975): 1840.

61. Jacqueline Rose Hott, "Updating Cherry Ames," *AJN* 77 (October 1977): 1582-1583.

62. Bonnie Bullough and Vern L. Bullough, "Sex Discrimination in Health Care," *Nursing Outlook* 23 (January 1975): 43.

63. Ruth Lubic Watson, "Developing Maternity Services Women Will Trust," *AJN* 75 (October 1975): 1687.

64. Joan E. Mulligan, "Professional Transition: Nurse to Nurse-Midwife," *Nursing Outlook* 24 (April 1976): 232-233.

65. Mary F. Kohnke, Ann Zimmern, and Jocelyn A. Greenidge, *Independent Nurse Practitioner* (Garden Grove, Ca.: Trainex Press, 1974), 2-3, 51-52.

66. Thelma M. Schorr, "Struggling for the Right to Do Right," *AJN* 80 (April 1980): 653.

67. Helen Ramirez and Elizabeth Washak, "Feminist Analysis: Illinois Nurse Midwife Situation," *Newsjournal* 3 (September 1985): 13.

68. ANA, *Facts, '80-'81,* 3, 39, 82; ANA, *Facts, '82-'83,* 1, 31, 68; Harold L. Hirsch and John M. Studner, "The Nurse Practitioner (NP) in Action: Patients' Friend, Physicians' Foe?" *Medical Trial Techniques Quarterly* (1985 annual): 38.

69. "Nurse-Practitioners - 53% More In 2 Years," *RN* 38 (August 1975): 5; Walter O. Spitzer, "The Nurse Practitioner Revisited: Slow Death of a Good Idea," *The New*

England Journal of Medicine 31 (19 April 1984): 1050; Scott Waters and Jean Arbeiter, "Nurse practitioners: How are they doing now?" *RN* 43 (October 1985): 39.

70. Harry A. Sultz et al., "A Decade of Change for Nurse Practitioners," *Nursing Outlook* 31 (May/June 1983): 141.

71. Eugene Levine, "What Do We Know About Nurse Practitioners," *AJN* 77 (November 1977): 1800.

72. Harry A. Sultz, et al., "A Decade of Change - Part III," *Nursing Outlook* 31 (September/October 1983): 268.

73. Martha Sturm White, "Psycholgical Characteristics of the Nurse Practitioner," *Nursing Outlook* 23 (March 1975): 162.

74. Sultz et al., "A Decade of Change - Part III," 269.

75. Loretta C. Ford, "Physicians' Assistant: Why, Who and How?" *AORN Journal* 15 (April 1972): 42-44.

76. Henry Silver and Loretta Ford, "The Pediatric Nurse Practitioner at Colorado," *AJN* 67 (July 1967): 1444; Henry K. Silver, Loretta C. Ford, and Lewis R. Day, "The Pediatric Nurse-Practitioner Program," *The Journal of the American Medical Association* 204 (22 April 1968): 299-300.

77. Kohnke, Zimmern, and Greenidge, *Independent Nurse Practitioner*, 28.

78. Kohnke, Zimmern, and Greenidge, *Independent Nurse Practitioner*, 22-26; Silver, Ford, and Day, "The Pediatric Nurse-Practitioner Program," 299; Harry A. Sultz, et al., "A Decade of Change - Part IV," *Nursing Outlook* 32 (May/June 1984): 162.

79. Darlene M. Trandel Korenchuk and Keith M. Trandel Korenchuk, "How State Laws Recognize Advanced Nursing Practice," *Nursing Outlook* 26 (November 1978): 713.

80. Ford, "Physicians' Assistant," 42.

81. Geraldene Felton, et al., "Nursing Entrepreneurs: A Success Story," *Nursing Outlook* 33 (November/December 1985): 278; "Midwives Tell Congressional Hearing Of Widespread Opposition by Doctors," *AJN* 81 (February 1981): 263.

82. Felton, et al., "Nursing Entrepreneurs," 278; Kohnke, Zimmern, and Greenidge, *Independent Nurse Practitioner*, 45; Sandra L. Robertson, "Letters," *AJN* 84 (May 1984): 595; Spitzer, "The Nurse Practitioner Revisited," 1050.

83. Kohnke, Zimmern, and Greenidge, *Independent Nurse Practitioner*, 104-105.

84. Ramirez and Washak, "Feminist Analysis," 13.

85. "Bellamy, NYSNA Seek Support for Expanded Practice," *AJN* 81 (December 1981): 2120, 2132; Jan R. Hartel, "Letters," *AJN* 74 (July 1974): 1242; "New Practice Act in Colorado Expands Definition of Nursing," *AJN* 80 (July 1980): 1261; "Primary Nurse Associate Recognized in Louisiana Law," *AJN* 81 (April 1981): 68; Smith, "Nursing Beyond the Crossroads," 543.

86. Kohnke, Zimmern, and Greenidge, *Independent Nurse Practitioner*, 107.

87. Bonnie Bullough, "The Current Phase in The Develoment Of Nurse Practice Acts," *Saint Louis University Law Journal* 28, no. 2 (1984): 381-385; David Weintraub, "A New Role for Nurses: The Nurse Practitioner," *Medical Trial Technique Quarterly* (1985 annual): 79.

88. "Inouye Bill S. 1702 Proposes Payment to Nurse-Midwives Under Medicaid/Medicare," *AJN* 77 (August 1977): 1241; "Inouye Bill Would Reimburse RNs Directly Under Medicare, Medicaid," *AJN* 77 (March 1977): 349; Sara Wriston, "Nurse Practitioner Reimbursement," *Journal of Health Politics, Policy, and Law* 6 (Fall 1981): 444.

89. Hurdis M. Griffith, "Strategies for Direct Third-Party Reimbursement For Nurses," *AJN* 82 (March 1982): 409; "Maryland Is First State to Require Third-Party Payment for Nurses," *AJN* 80 (January 1980): 7.

90. Sarah D. Cohn, "Survey of Legislation on Third Party Reimbursement for Nurses," *Law, Medicine, and Health Care* 11 (December 1983): 260; "N.J. Nurse Entrepreneurs Now Eligible For 3rd-Party Reimbursement," *AJN* 84 (March 1984): 377; "NPs Battle To Expand Practice: Connecticut Gets Reimbursement," *AJN* 84 (November 1984): 1424.

91. Griffith, "Strategies for Direct Third-Party Reimbursement," 409-410; "Nurse Practitioners Testify," *AJN* 74 (July 1974): 1214.

92. Cammie O'Shaughessy, "Diary Of An Angry Nurse-Practitioner," *AJN* 76 (July 1976): 1166-1168; Donna L. Wong, "Private Practice - At a Price," *Nursing Outlook* 25 (April 1977): 258.

93. "D.C. CNMs, NPs Have High Hopes For Admitting Privileges," *AJN* 83 (November 1983): 1607, 1616; "D.C. Oks Staff Privileges For CNMs, NPs," *AJN* 84 (January 1984): 123; Michael Rose, "Laying Siege To Hospital Privileges," *AJN* 84 (May 1984): 615.

94. "JCAH Is Weighing Wider Access To Staff Privileges in Hospitals," *AJN* 83 (September 1983): 1260; Karen Mitchell, "The Death of the Goose That Laid the Golden Egg," *Pediatric Nursing* 10 (March/April 1984): 101; "Non-MDs Can Join Medical Staffs, Says JCAH," *AJN* 84 (March 1984): 382.

95. Evans, *Personal Politics*, 15-21; Kessler-Harris, *Out to Work*, 314-315.

96. Virginia Cleland, "To End Sex Discrimination," *Nursing Clinics of North America* 9 (September 1974): 565.

97. "ANA Institutes Complaint Of Salary Discrimination By Pittsburgh University," *AJN* 77 (September 1977): 1394; "After Five Years, Sex Discrimination Suit Comes to Court," *AJN* 79 (June 1979): 1040; "B.U. Nursing Faculty Claims Discrimination," *AJN* 74 (July 1974): 1209; "High Court Action Frees Salary Data in Sex-Bias Suit," *AJN* 81 (December 1981): 2117, 2220; "Nursing School Faculty Charges Discrimination in Class Action Suit," *AJN* 74 (April 1974): 602.

98. "ANA Charges Pension Fund and Three Universities with Sex Discrimination," *AJN* 73 (April 1973): 586; "ANA Files Charges of Sex Discrimination," *Nursing Outlook* 21 (May 1973): 278; Cleland, "To End Sex Discrimination," 568; "EEOC Upholds Charges of Sex Discrimination in University Pensions," *AJN* 74 (September 1974): 1557.

99. ANA, *Facts, '80-'81,* 3, 39, 82; ANA, *Facts, '82-'83,* 1, 31, 68.

100. Nancy J. Brent, "The Nurse Practitioner After Sermchief And Fein: Smooth Sailing Or Rough Waters?" *Valparaiso University Law Review* 21 (Winter 1987): 230-233; Margaret L. Hunter, "These nurses weren't practicing medicine after all," *RN* 47 (January 1984): 69; Mary B. Mallison, "A Tale Of Two Coalitions," *AJN* 84 (January 1984): 7; "Missouri NPs Win Appeal in Medical Practicesuit," *AJN* 84 (January 1984): 111, 132; "NPs Appeal Ruling Limiting Practice in FP Clinics," *AJN* 83 (March 1983): 358, 360.

101. "Brent, The Nurse Practitioner," 230-233; Hunter, "These nurses," 69; Mallison, "A Tale Of Two Coalitions," 7; "Missouri NPs Win Appeal," 111, 132.

102. "Missouri NPs Win Appeal," 132.

103. Mallison, "A Tale Of Two Coalitions," 7.

104. "FTC: Insurance Cannot Be Withheld From MDs Who Work with CNMs," *AJN* 83 (August 1983): 1123; Elisabeth Hyde, "Territorial Imperatives in Health Care," *Nursing Outlook* 32 (May/June 1984): 136; "Nashville nurse-midwives," *AJN* 83 (January 1983): 12; "Nashville Nurse Midwives Fight for Hospital Privileges," *AJN* 80 (October 1980): 1722; "Nurse-Midwives Sue Nashville Doctors," *AJN* 82 (June 1982): 914; Donna M. Peizer, "A Social and Legal Analysis of the Independent Practice of Midwifery," *Berkeley Women's Law Journal* 2 (Fall 1986): 202-204; "Tennessee's ACOG Reiterates Stand In Midwife Tussle," *AJN* 81 (April 1981): 673, 681.

105. "Nurse-Midwives Sue," 914.

106. Hyde, "Territorial Imperatives," 137.

107. Blum, *Between Feminism and Labor,* 2.

108. Madalon Amenta, "Nurses' NOW: A Model of Worksite Organizing" (paper presented at the Women's Caucus, American Public Health Association Meeting, Washington, D.C., 31 October 1977), 1; Blum, *Between Feminism and Labor,* 185.

109. Blum, *Between Feminism and Labor,* 106.

110. JoAnn Ashley, "Power in Structured Misogyny: Implications for the Politics of Care," *ANS* 2 (April 1980): 18-19.

111. Vincent O'Neal, "You really are underpaid," *RN* 42 (May 1979): 79.

112. "California Decrees Comparable Worth Of Women's Work," *AJN* 81 (November 1981): 1984.

113. Blum, *Between Feminism and Labor,* 51-52; O'Neal, "You really are underpaid," 2 "Salaries Don't Match RN Responsibilities, Jacox Tells EEOC," *AJN* 80 (July 1980): 1242; "Women Underpaid EEOC Is Told; Report Backs 'Comparable Worth,' " *AJN* 81 (November 1981): 1967.

114. "ANA Named to Board Of New Coalition On Pay Equity," *AJN* 81 (January 1981): 7.

115. "Continued Support for Equal Rights," 4; "Pay Equity, Competition, Values To Be Probed at ANA Convention," *AJN* 82 (May 1982): 746; "Report of the Perspec-

tives Committee," *1983 Business Book, NLN Biennial Convention, Philadelphia, June 1-4, 1983,* NLN Headquarters, New York, 33.

116. Patricia S. Chaney, "Protest," *Nursing 77* 7 (February 1977): 30-33; "Comparing Man/Woman Pay, Nurses Bring Charges," *AJN* 75 (July 1975): 1104; "Denver Nurses Charge Sex Discrimination in Pay Scales," *AJN* 77 (February 1977): 181, 183; Thelma M. Schorr, "It's Happening in Denver," *AJN* 78 (July 1978): 1187.

117. "ANA Helps Fund Sex-Discrimination Case," *AJN* 76 (January 1976): 137; Chaney, "Protest," 33; "Comparing Man/Woman Pay," 104; "Cookbook Raises Funds For Denver Lawsuit," *AJN* 77 (September 1977): 1384.

118. Bonnie Bullough, "The Struggle For Women's Rights in Denver: A Personal Account," *Nursing Outlook* 26 (September 1978): 567.

119. Lois O'Brien Friss, "Work Force Policy Perspectives: Registered Nurses," *Journal of Health Politics, Policy, and Law* 5 (Winter 1981): 701-705; Schorr, "It's Happening in Denver," 1187; Margretta Styles, "The Uphill Battle for Comparable Worth," *Nursing Outlook* 33 (May/June 1985): 129.

120. "Denver Nurses File Appeal in Sex Bias Suit Lost in 1978," *AJN* 79 (February 1979): 206; "Denver RNs Appeal Judicial Decision On Pay-Scale Suit," *AJN* 78 (June 1978): 957; NURSE, Inc. Plans Supreme Court Appeal," *AJN* 80 (September 1980): 1546; "Supreme Court Declines to Hear NURSE, Inc. Case," *AJN* 80 (December 1980): 2127; "Review of Nurses' Pay Suit Denied by Supreme Court," *Nursing Outlook* 81 (January 1981): 29.

121. Blum, *Between Feminism and Labor,* 50-52.

122. "Comp Worth Study: 'Nurses Really Underpaid,' " *AJN* 84 (February 1984): 256-257; Nancy E. Dowd, "The Metamorphosis Of Comparable Worth," *Suffolk University Law Review* 20 (Winter 1986): 852; "Illinois RNs Win Appeal in Wage-Bias Suit," *AJN* 86 (May 1986): 608; Lois R. Lupica, "Pay Equity - a 'Cockamamie' Idea: The Future of Health Care May Depend Upon It," *American Journal Of Law & Medicine* 13, no. 4 (1988): 611-612; Lawrence D. MacLachlan, "Letters," *Nursing Outlook* 34 (March/April 1986): 104; "Wisconsin RNs Win Comparable Worth Fight," *1199 News* 19 (August-September 1984): 10.

123. Edith Barnett, interview by author, tape recording, 26 February 1991, Washington, D.C; " 'Historic' Settlement Reached in PNA's Sex Discrimination Lawsuit," 5 May 1987, Dorothy M. Novello Memorial Library, The Pennsylvania Nurses Association, Harrisburg, Pennsylvania; Subjects #9 and #17.

124. "Madison Public Health RNs' Settle Contract; File Sex Discrimination Complaint with EEOC," *AJN* 77 (July 1977): 1096; Seymour Mokskowitz, "Pay Equity And American Nurses: A Legal Analysis," *St. Louis University Law Journal* 27 (November 1983): 828-831; "Wisconsin RNs," 10.

125. "ANA Votes Federation," 1250; Mary B. Mallison, "Deciding What You're Worth," *AJN* 83 (June 1983): 875; "U/Georgia NPs Stung By Court's Decision On Pay-Equity Charge," *AJN* 85 (July 1985): 832.

126. "Action on Resolutions," *Convention Report, 1986,* American Federation of Teachers, AFL-CIO, Sixty-Ninth Convention, Grand Ballroom, Hyatt Regency, Chi-

cago, Illinois, 3-8 July, 1986, New York State School of Industrial and Labor Relations, Martin P. Catherwood Library, Labor-Management Documentation Center, Cornell University, 22-23; "AFSCME Scrapbook," *Public Employee* 45 (January 1980): 15; "AFSCME Women's Conference Focuses on Pay Equity and Politics," *Public Employee* 47 (November-December 1983): 10; "Committees Study Clerical, Professional Needs," *Public Employee* 45 (January 1980): 13; "Contract Crunch for 13,000 Members," *1199 News* 20 (June-July 1985): 3; "Only Unions Can Bring Women's Wages On Par With Men's," *Service Employee* 40 (December 1980): 6-7; William Lucy, "National Commission on Working Women Deserves Our Full Support," *Public Employee* 45 (April 1980): 11; "Pay Equity: The Economic Issue of the 80's,' " *Public Employee* 44 (November 1979): 5; "Report of the IEB, *18th International Convention, 13-17 May 1984, Dearborn, Michigan, Service Employees Official Proceedings,* New York State School of Industrial and Labor Relations, Martin P. Catherwood Library, Labor-Management Documentation Center, Cornell University, xv, xx; "Washington RNs Ask Lawmakers To Fund Salary Hike For Women," *AJN* 85 (March 1985): 317; "What's This 'Pay Equity,' " *Service Employee* 41 (October 1981): 12.

127. "Partial Report of the Resolution Committee," *AFSCME Proceedings of the 27th International Convention,* Chicago, Illinois, 23-27 June 1986, New York State School of Industrial and Labor Relations, Martin P. Catherwood Library, Labor-Management Documentation Center, Cornell University, 86.

128. Lupica, "Pay Equity," 611-612, 617.

129. Richard P. Stober, "Women Are Paid Less Than Men. Solution? Comparable Worth!" *The Pennsylvania Nurse* 39 (May 1984): 9.

130. "Nurses Back On Job," 8; "OUSE Members Ratify New COP Agreement, Six to One," *The Pennsylvania Nurse* 38 (August 1983): 15; "Pennsylvania Will Study 'Comparable Worth' Of Its RNs," *AJN* 83 (October 1983): 1474; Purcell, "Nurses Strike," 1; Subjects #9 and #17.

131. Blum, *Between Feminism and Labor,* 54-91; Judy L. Brett, "How Much Is A Nurse's Job Really Worth?" *AJN* 83 (June 1983): 881; Margaret Weingard, "Establishing Comparable Worth Through Job Evaluation," *Nursing Outlook* 32 (March/April 1984): 113.

132. Blum, *Between Feminism and Labor,* 106-123; "Resolute Contra Costa RNs Show How To Win A Comp. Worth Raise," *AJN* 85 (March 1985): 317.

133. Blum, *Between Feminism and Labor,* 105-107.

134. Barnett interview; Edith Barnett, "PNA Memorandum in Support of EEOC Charges," Dorothy M. Novello Memorial Library, The Pennsylvania Nurses Association, Harrisburg, Pennsylvania; Subject #9.

135. "San Jose R.N.s Seek Raise to $30,000 in Contract Talks," *AJN* 81 (November 1981): 1968.

136. "Steinem Supports RNs," *AJN* 82 (May 1982): 745; "Steinem Walks the Line with San Jose RNs," *AJN* 82 (May 1982): 750.

137. Blum, *Between Feminism and Labor,* 117.

138. "AHA's New Data Shed Light On Hospital Staffing," *AJN* 84 (June 1984): 809; "Nurses Notebook," *Nursing 84* 14 (January 1984): 80; "One in Three Hospitals Claim Nursing Shortage," *The Pennsylvania Nurse* 38 (February 1984): 10.

139. Matt Clark, et al., "Nurses: Few and Fatigued," *Newsweek,* 29 June 1987, 59.

140. "Recruiters Rebound As Shortage Escalates," *AJN* 86 (September 1986): 1054.

141. "R.N.s' with Graduate Degrees Are Scarce; Report Dispells Myth About Causes of Shortage," *The Pennsylvania Nurse* 38 (March 1983): 5.

142. "Job prospects bright for nurses with degrees," *RN* 46 (November 1984): 12.

143. "Demand For Critical Care Nurses Keeps Soaring: Crunch Is Reaching Medical-Surgical Units, Too," *AJN* 86 (September 1986): 1052; "RN Shortages Sprout in Reagan's Backyard," *AJN* 86 (November 1986): 1285; "With ICUs Filling Up, Hospitals Are Searching High And Low For More Critical Care Nurses," *AJN* 81 (November 1981): 1970.

144. Clark, et al., "Nurses: Few and Fatigued," 59; Kenneth Green, "Nurses For The Future: What The Freshmen Tell Us," *AJN* 87 (December 1987): 1610-1611; "Kaiser Calls On Legislators For Solution To RN Shortages," *AJN* 86 (December 1986): 1419.

145. Lucie S. Kelly, "A Matter Of Choices," *Nursing Outlook* 32 (September/October 1984): 249.

146. Peter T. Kilborn, "Nurses Get V.I.P. Treatment, Easing Shortage," *New York Times,* 1 May 1990, 1.

147. Thelma M. Schorr, "Focus on the Nurse Shortage," *AJN* 80 (September 1980): 1587.

148. Philip A. Kalisch and Beatrice J. Kalisch, "The Nurse Shortage, the Present, and the Congress," *Nursing Forum* 19, no. 2 (1980): 142.

149. Karen Davis, "Non-Nursing Functions: Our Readers Respond," *AJN* 82 (December 1982): 1857, 1860.

150. "News," *AJN* 86 (November 1986): 1297.

151. "Alabama Studies Cite Underpaid, Undervalued RNs," *AJN* 81 (December 1981): 2136; "Job Disatisfaction Causes R.N. Shortage, Texas Study Shows," *AJN* 80 (September 1980): 1527.

152. Ann L. Steck, "The Nursing Shortage: An Optimistic View," *Nursing Outlook* 29 (May 1981): 302.

153. Kelly, "A Matter Of Choices," 249.

154. Clark, et al., "Nurses: Few and Fatigued," 61; Green, "What The Freshmen Tell Us," 1612; Sandra Mary Hillman, "The Effects Of College Going Women's Current Values And Attitudes On The Decline in Enrollments To Baccalaureate Programs in Nursing," (Ph.D. dissertation, Boston College, 1983), 56, 88, 104.

155. "Bill to Amend NLRA Definition of Supervisor Is Introduced," *AJN* 78 (January 1978): 7; "Landmark Ruling: VA Head Nurses Are Not Supervisors," *AJN* 80

(December 1980): 2125; "New Jersey RN Barbara Schelling Knows What Being a 'Supervisor' Can Mean," *AJN* 78 (January 1978): 21; " 'Supervisor' Language Is Clarified in Civil Service Act," *AJN* 78 (December 1978): 2001.

156. "... And One That Did," *Service Employee* 31 (May 1980): 12; Catherine S. Ballman, "Union Busters," *AJN* 85 (September 1985): 963-966; "New Mexico Election A Victory for Workers and Their Community," *1199 News* 21 (January 1986): 10; "Partial Report of the Organizing Committee," *AFSCME, Proceedings of the 25th International Convention*, Atlantic City, N.J., 1982, New York State School of Industrial and Labor Relations, Martin P. Catherwood Library, Labor-Management Documentation Center, Cornell University, 156-157; "Union-Busting Discussed at RN Workshop," *1199 News* 17 (January 1982): 19.

157. Rita E. Numeroff and Michael N. Abrams, "Collective bargaining among nurses: current issues and future prospects," *Health Care Management Review* 9 (Spring 1984): 65; "Prop. 13 Said to Be Causing Shortages in California Services," *AJN* 78 (December 1978): 2002, 2026, 2032; Pettengill, "Multilateral Collective Bargaining," 278-279; Thelma M. Schorr, "Cost, Not Care, Containment," *AJN* 77 (July 1977): 1129; "SNAs Sue Rate Commissions For Blocking Wage Increases," *AJN* 83 (November 1983): 1611.

158. Waters and Arbeiter, "Nurse practitioners," 41.

159. Jerry L. Weston, "Whither the 'Nurse' in Nurse Practitioner," *Nursing Outlook* 23 (March 1975): 169.

160. Wriston, "Nurse Practitioner Reimbursement," 451-456.

161. Bonnie Bullough, "Legal Restrictions as a Barrier to Nurse Practitioner Role Development," *Pediatric Nursing* 10 (November/December 1984): 439-441.

162. "Nurse Practitioners Fight Moves To Restrict Their Practices," *AJN* 78 (August 1978): 1285, 1308, 1310; "State Board Regulations for NPs Become Legal Issue in Two States," *AJN* 81 (August 1981): 1432-1433.

163. "NP Prescribing Privileges Attacked in Oregon," *AJN* 81 (April 1981): 653.

164. "MDs' Suit Against Louisiana Board Dismissed by Judge," *AJN* 82 (March 1982): 376; "State Board Regulations," 1432-1433; "Texas Judge Backs Nursing Board's Regulation of NPs," *AJN* 83 (Feburary 1983): 202.

165. "University of Washington Faculty Appeals Sex Discrimination Decision," *AJN* 79 (September 1979): 1508.

166. Cleland, "To End Sex Discrimination," 566.

167. Lupica, "Pay Equity," 612.

168. Blum, *Between Feminism and Labor*, 178, 120-121.

169. Donna Newberry, "Letters," *AJN* 82 (August 1982): 1198.

170. Subject #4.

CHAPTER 6:

The Obstacles to Feminism

In her 1975 article, "Nursing and Early Feminism," JoAnn Ashley exhibited great optimism about her profession's future. Pointing to such developments as *ANA v. TIAA* and the formation of Nurses NOW, Ashley believed nurses had the power to eradicate sexism and win fair salaries and autonomy. Although nurses had dealt with male chauvinism, gender stereotyping, and discrimination since the profession's beginnings, Ashley now saw "a brighter side on the horizon."[1]

Ashley's vision, however, proved to be premature. Nurses did achieve notable successes during the 1970s and 1980s. But they also encountered problems in their fight for equality. R.N.s had difficulty implementing strategies such as collective bargaining, comparable worth, and third-party reimbursement. Courts did not always side with nurses even in the cases where blatant discrimination had occurred.

Nursing, along with the larger women's movement, also faced political challenges. The conservative backlash of the 1970s and 1980s hurt feminists of all backgrounds and strands. As conservative candidates won political offices, the women's movement came under attack. State and federal governments deregulated business and dismantled social programs. President Ronald Reagan's administration, for example, cut federal daycare subsidies, dismantled the existing civil rights machinery, and appointed conservatives to the EEOC and NLRB.[2] In 1984 the chair of the Civil Rights Commission, a Reagan appointee, called pay equity " 'the looniest idea since Looney Tunes.' "[3] Social conservatives such as Phyllis Schafly, who deplored the breakdown of traditional gender roles, fought the Equal Rights Amendment and reproductive choice. They prevented ERA ratification in 1982 and pressured Congress to withold funding for abortions. Their successes pointed out both the political strength of this neo-conservative movement and the increasingly unfavorable climate in which feminists operated.[4]

Nurses, however, experienced several additional obstacles. During the 1970s the women's movement largely ignored nursing and other feminized professions. Groups such as NOW concentrated their energies instead on females in male-dominated occupations. Feminists also encountered difficulties in the nursing press. While the ANA's and NLN's organs — the *AJN* and *Nursing Outlook* — supported the women's movement, other publications took a less positive stance. Those periodicals which portrayed "women's libbers" as strident, man-hating bra-burners gave feminist R.N.s an unflattering image and hampered their attempts to communicate with sympathetic colleagues. This negative coverage also alienated potential allies. Finally, nurses themselves were divided over the women's movement. Traditionalist R.N.s held beliefs in direct opposition to those of their feminist coworkers. Other nurses adopted a mixture of feminist and more conventional attitudes. Personal characteristics and professional experiences heavily influenced where individuals stood on the feminist-traditionalist continuum.

Studying nursing has revealed a great deal about the experiences and beliefs of women in postwar America. It has explained the increased labor force participation of married females; the impact of college education upon baby boomers; and the goals, tactics, and strands of the re-emerging women's movement. Examining the obstacles faced by feminst nurses and the divisions within the profession likewise illuminates much about contemporary U.S. society. In particular it helps explain the backlash against feminism and why so many American women, well into the 1980s, found the movement threatening.

During the early 1970s, however, feminist nurses' biggest challenge seemed to be acceptance by the larger women's movement. In their eagerness to break down barriers in male-dominated fields, liberal feminist organizations such as NOW paid little attention to females in traditional jobs. At times the women's movement displayed great insensitivity towards R.N.s. It seemed ignorant of both the potential for organizing nurses and the profession's social importance. Nurses felt these slights keenly. In 1975 Elizabeth Harding, a San Francisco nursing professor, astutely analyzed the problem.

> It is important that women who wish to be doctors be allowed that alternative; however, the emphasis conveys a negative message to many other women health workers.

First, it fails to address itself to a potentially strong force in the health system - the 80 percent of all health workers who are women but not doctors. By ignoring them, the women's movement is alienating the majority of health workers. Their attitude implies that to be "liberated," these women must become doctors.... The women's movement has accepted the male standard of judging people by the power they hold....

Second, encouraging women to be doctors is of little help to other women health workers.... These workers need the support, help, and experience of the women's movement, and they are not getting it. Third, this physician-centered attitude demonstrates the inability of the women's movement to deal positively with those aspects of society that are labeled "feminine" or "women's work."[5]

Two University of Wisconsin professors, writing in 1978, agreed with this assessment. They observed,

many feminist groups view nursing as the ultimate expression of the denigration of women.... Many feminist leaders on our own campus hold this view....[6]

Even NOW founder, Betty Friedan, admitted in a 1981 interview that the women's movement had ignored nurses.[7]

By the late 1970s and early 1980s feminist groups were more likely to address issues such as pay equity and childcare, which were of concern to more typical female workers.[8] Still, the alliance between nursing and the women's movement remained fragile. In 1981 two New York City R.N.s expressed shock at the negative images of nurses portrayed in local NOW literature.[9] Four years later a group of nurse-authors noted that feminists still saw nursing "as one of the ultimate female ghettos from which women should be encouraged to escape."[10]

Even Nurses NOW encountered discrimination within the women's movement. In fact NOW's tactlessness at its 1973 convention actually spurred the nurses to organize. R.N.s attending this meeting were appalled when NOW president, Karen DeCrow, introduced Wilma Scott Heide as "a former nurse who went on up from there." Their fury prompted the first meeting of the Nurses NOW core group and the decision to organize as an occupational task force.[11] Even with NOW's official support, nurses had difficulty changing the attitudes of other feminists. Well into the 1970s activists in Pittsburgh, Nurses NOW's headquarters, distributed posters which read "Why A Nurse, Not A Doctor?"[12] This insensitivity alienated potential nurse-recruits and left bitterness in its wake.

Allying with larger women's groups, then, proved to be difficult for nurses. Feminist R.N.s, therefore, looked for support from their professional associations and the organizations' official publications. From the early 1970s onward, articles such as Ashley's "About Power in Nursing" and Cleland's "Sex Discrimination" had analyzed nursing's problems from a feminist perspective. These pieces also offered solutions for reforming the health care patriarchy. The *AJN* and *Nursing Outlook* had publicized the formation of Nurses NOW, raised legal funds for Denver litigants, and urged nurses to lobby for the ERA.

Certain elements within the professional press, however, took a different approach and had a negative impact upon the efforts of feminist nurses. *RN*, a journal owned by a subsidiary of the medical equipment company Litton Industries, belittled and poked fun at the women's movement. In 1972, for example, editor Richard F. Newcomb, hailed the assignment of the first female naval officer to sea duty with the following memo.

> What an historic moment! The first woman in history to make the real, seagoing Navy. And what luck! She was just in time for a six-week wintertime patrol in the North Pacific! There is nothing quite so attractive as the North Pacific - so much water, so much space, so much - er, nothing. But in the wintertime, oh what special attractions — that wind, so strong, so relentless, so penetrating. And nothing like taking it full force on the midnight-to-4 A.M. watch on the forecastle, which is what the newest ensign is likely to draw.
>
> So have a nice cruise, Ensign Mary Lou McCarthy, and don't worry about the midwatch. You'll get off it eventually and not *all* cruises are 42 days out of sight of land.
>
> Only kidding, of course, but I guess the moral might be: Before you get liberated, be sure you know what you're getting liberated to.
>
> Aside: Come to think of it, why *do* they call ships "she?" Isn't that discriminatory against men?[13]

RN did not publish a serious analysis of sex discrimination in nursing until 1979. It disregarded Nurses NOW until 1978, four years after NOW formally chartered the group.[14]

Nursing, a skill journal published by Intermed Communications, engaged in similar barbs. After a 1973 interview with two members of the feminist group, Nurses for Political Action, a staff writer referred to the women's movement as "glib lib."[15] One year later the journal attempted to link nurse-activists with the radical feminists portrayed in the popular media. In an article which discussed nurses' strikes, one author referred to union members as women who might "burn their caps in protest."[16] Even after *RN* modified its coverage, *Nursing* did not discuss professional issues in feminist terms.

Sensationalized press coverage was nothing new for feminists. The national media had already played up the antics of radical "guerilla theater" groups such as SCUM (Society for Cutting Up Men) which burned bras and disrupted bridal fairs. This coverage made extremely good copy. But it had also antagonized much of the American public. In the popular mindset "women's libbers" had become aggressive, man-hating, bra-burning Amazons.[17]

As was true for feminists in the wider society, negative portrayals of the women's movement had important consequences for nurses. *RN* and *Nursing* were popular publications, with circulations much larger than that of either the *AJN* or *Nursing Outlook*.[18] Thus their failure to treat the movement in a positive manner cost nurse-feminists potential allies. For one thing dissatisfied R.N.s, who read this segment of the press, were unlikely to learn about feminist nursing groups or issues such as the ERA. Furthermore, many nurses who read the popular journals undoubtedly came to perceive feminists as strident, bitter extremists. Nurses NOW founders, for example, had difficulty convincing potential members that they were not "radicals who wanted to burn down the hospital."[19] Other nurse-activists had similar experiences. A PNA labor organizer recalled that in the 1970s even ardent unionists saw feminists as bra-burners and man-haters.[20] One local unit leader remembered that her coworkers believed "women's libbers" were all "gays, queers, and lesbians."[21]

Nursing, then, was a profession divided over the women's movement. These divisions went well beyond the differences among the various strands of feminists. Traditionalist nurses reacted to talk of women's equality and liberation with horror. They saw feminism as a philosophy which degraded women's natural, time-honored roles, weakened the family, and led to narcissism. Other nurses took a more middle-of-the-road approach. They supported the economic planks of the feminist platform such as pay equity. But they did not totally reject the sexual division of labor, either. Middle-roaders also felt uncomfortable with the feminist label and thus hesitated to completely identify themselves with the women's movement. While negative media coverage played a role in creating these rifts, it was not the only, nor even the most significant, factor which split the profession. Nurses' educational backgrounds, work histories, ages, and other personal and professional characteristics had a major impact on how they perceived the women's movement.

As mentioned earlier, feminist nurses, no matter what their strand, represented a distinct group within nursing. These women were college-educated, career-committed, active in professional organizations, and employed in what were considered elite specialities. An analysis of the careers of twenty feminist nursing leaders, while by no means exhaustive, illustrates how certain personal characteristics and life experiences propelled women towards feminism (See Appendix 1).

Nursing leaders, allied with the women's movement between 1970-1986, engaged in a variety of activities designed to promote change. Many wrote consciousness-raising articles for the professional press, and participated in seminars and programs on feminism. Nurse-journalists — notably *AJN* editors Barbara Schutt, Thelma Schorr, and Mary Mallison, and *Nursing Outlook's* Edith Patton Lewis, Jeanne Fonesca, and Penny McCarthy — used their publications to educate R.N.s about the movement. Professional association officers such as the ANA's Eunice Cole, Barbara Nichols, and Anne Zimmerman, lobbied and testified for feminist agenda items such as the ERA and equal pay legislation.[22] No matter what form their participation took, these leaders shared similarities in terms of education, occupation, professional affiliations, and nursing specialities.

Eighty percent of these women had been born prior to 1940, but their lives were distinctly different from their age-mates in nursing's rank-and-file. All had been employed continuously over their lifetimes. All had obtained at least a BSN. Sixteen (eighty percent) held masters degrees and ten (fifty percent) had earned a Ph.D. or Ed.D. Eleven (fifty-five percent) worked as college professors and deans of nursing, while six (thirty percent) were editors of nursing journals. One was a self-employed home health care consultant, another the executive director of a state nursing association. One worked in hospital administration at the onset of the 1970s, but left that position for a job on an SNA staff in 1982. Seven (thirty-five percent) had experience in psychiatric nursing and an additional five (twenty-five percent) had worked in either nursing administration or public health. Ninety percent were active in the ANA or an SNA, forty percent were fellows in the American Academy of Nursing (FAAN), and thirty percent belonged to the NLN.

These experiences promoted feminist perspectives in several ways. Like the college-educated nurses discussed in Chapter 3, these leaders learned new values and skills, developed a strong sense of professionalism, and grew impatient with the status quo. As long-term wage earners and ambitious professionals, they had experienced sexism. Thus the feminist critique of U.S. society seemed applicable to their own lives. This enabled them to draw parallels between the plight of nurses in the health care system and the position of women in U.S. society. Furthermore, since many of them were employed in relatively autonomous settings, they exhibited less subservience than nurses who worked directly under physicians.[23] Participation in professional associations allowed them to share their frustrations, formulate solutions, and engage in collective action.

Those employed in the university faced problems which clearly opened their eyes to sexism. Academic nurses held credentials and levels of responsibility identical to those of their male colleagues. As they sought funding for nursing departments and applied for promotion and tenure, they encountered sex discrimination. Virginia Cleland's 1971 complaints were echoed throughout the decade by other nurse-professors.[24] They grumbled about lower salaries and higher contact hours, arguing that nursing departments received unfair treatment because their faculty members were women.[25] University-employed nurses also believed their departments suffered from low prestige within the male-dominated academy.[26] One educator complained to Edith Patton Lewis in 1974 that,

> the nursing school dean and the nursing school itself are just second-class citizens. My budget is the first to be cut, my faculty the last to get professorships. An adequate library? Funds and facilities for research? Forget it![27]

Employment in colleges and universities, therefore, provided unique opportunities for consciousness-raising, experiences denied nurses who worked in other settings.

Employment and research in the psychiatric field also made R.N.s receptive to feminism. For one thing, psychiatric nurses, like educators, had considerable autonomy from male physicians and administrators.[28] Secondly, because of what they saw in their practices and research data, many became interested specifically in the emotional development and psychology of women.[29] Psychiatric nurses came to believe that much of female neuroses and depression resulted from male-defined standards of femininity and society's refusal to value women's talents and goals.[30] They further stated that male therapists, operating out of patriarchal value systems, harmed female patients. Several practitioners were able to document cases where feminist-centered treatment facilitated recovery.[31]

Rank-and-file nurses who identified with the women's movement exhibited many of these same characteristics. Interviews conducted with eighteen feminist nurses reveal important links among education, professional experiences, family characteristics, age, and opinions about feminism (See Figure 14).[32] These women, activists from Nurses NOW and the Pennsylvania Nurses Association, were identified by the author through both organizational literature and snowball interview techniques. These nurses defined themselves as feminists, supported the Equal Rights Amendment, and advocated legalized abortion. All championed pay equity and nurses' right to unionize. Ten (fifty-six percent) had, in fact, been local unit officers or organizers. Two women had been heavily involved in PNA's 1987 lawsuit against the Commonwealth.

Like the leaders discussed above, the feminist rank-and-file represented the highly educated, career-oriented, activist segment of the profession. They also came from the postwar, baby boom generation. Sixteen (eighty-nine percent) had been born after 1940. All had worked in nursing for at least ten years and fourteen (seventy-eight percent) had been employed for over twenty. Many worked in autonomous settings. Only one (five percent) had worked continuously as a hospital general duty nurse.[33] Seven (thirty-nine percent) were employed in administration, education, and public health.[34] Two (eleven percent) worked, for at least part of their careers, as professional association officials.[35] Five (twenty-eight percent) were self-employed nursing consultants and three (seventeen percent) worked in hospitals as clinical specialists.[36] These nurses were also college-educated. All possessed a BSN. Seventy-eight percent held masters degrees and eleven percent had earned Ph.D.s. All were past or present ANA members and six (thirty-three percent) belonged to nursing sororities or specialty organizations.[37]

Rank-and-file feminists were either self-supporting or had experienced the strains of combining paid employment and family life. Fifty-five percent had been married only once. Eleven percent had never married, while seventeen percent were divorced. Another seventeen percent had divorced and remarried. Fifty-five percent had one or two children and seventeen percent had three or four. Twenty-eight percent were childless. All the mothers in the sample had worked while their children were young. Some cited financial need, others worked for intellectual stimulation or a combination of factors. All but one of the divorced women supported children. One woman financially contributed to her aged parents and a disabled sibling.[38]

FIGURE 14: PERSONAL CHARACTERISTICS OF 48 NURSES[a]
(Percentage in each category)[b]

	Feminist n=18	Traditionalist n=8	Middle-Road n=22
Year of Birth			
Before 1940	11	25	23
After 1940	89	75	77
Education			
Diploma	0	75	54
B.S.N.	11	12.5	32
M.S.N/Ph.D.	89	12.5	14
Occupation			
Staff Nurse	5	25	54
Homemaker	0	75	23
Other	95	0	23
Yrs. Employed			
0-5	0	63	5
5-10	0	13	18
10-15	11	12	18
15-20	11	0	41
20 or More	78	12	18
Prof. Org.			
ANA	100	12.5	64
Speciality	33	12.5	23
Marital Status			
Never Married	11	12.5	4
First Marriage	55	75	86
Widowed	0	12.5	5
Divorced	17	0	5
Remarried	17	0	0
Children			
0	28	12.5	10
1-2	55	25	45
3-4	17	50	36
5-6	0	12.5	9

[a.] *Source:* Interview Subject Database.

[b.] *Note:* Numbers in vertical columns will equal one hundred with the exception of Prof. Org. Many of the interview subjects belonged to more than one organization while others had no professional memberships.

Because of their experiences at college, home, the work place, and the nursing association, these women became feminists. They saw themselves as professionals and felt the sting of gender discrimination. They also had access to colleagues, theories, and tactics which challenged the sex hierarchy. They perceived the women's movement as a means of helping females acquire "their basic human rights."[39] Feminism, for them, helped women achieve their potentials, have independent lives, and acquire self-esteem.[40] Pay equity and unionization were ways to raise the issue of discrimination, teach females assertiveness, and redress women's historically low wages.[41]

These R.N.s believed that, aside from obvious anatomical disparities, no significant differences existed between males and females. As one woman observed, "It never occurred to me that I couldn't do what men do."[42] Feminist nurses therefore argued that equal opportunity was essential. All asserted their right to a career and completely rejected the sexual division of labor. The married feminists lived within egalitarian families. One remarked, "I stand up for my rights at home. In my household, responsibilities are shared equally."[43] The childless nurses consciously decided to forgo parenthood, while the mothers tended to take maternity leaves and return rather quickly to paid labor.[44] Feminist mothers worked for professional and personal reasons as well as for economic ones. One woman, reflecting on her return to work after the birth of her second child, remembered, "I wanted to be able to talk about something besides Pampers."[45]

These nurses also tended to support the larger, feminist platform. They saw the Equal Rights Amendment, for example, as a way to guarantee female equality. Several had participated in pro-ERA activities during the 1970s and early 1980s.[46] All feminist respondents strongly supported a woman's right to a safe and legal abortion. They perceived an unwanted pregnancy as a problem which unfairly burdened the female half of a sexual partnership. Thus one interview subject, concerned about ending the sexual division of labor in the family, saw abortion as a way of challenging the patriarchy.[47] Reproductive choice also enabled women to "be self-determining in matters related to their health and well-being."[48]

The philosophy outlined above, however, was not the only position taken by R.N.s. Eight traditionalist and twenty-two middle-road interview subjects had major differences with feminists. Traditionalists and middle-roaders were members of Birthright, Pennsylvanians for Human Life, and the PNA. Like feminist subjects, they were identified through association literature and snowball interviews. Although this sample is admitedly small, the interviews revealed important disagreements among various groups of nurses. Traditionalists and middle-roaders differed with feminists on gender roles, the women's movement, and, in the case of traditionalists, professional issues such as pay equity and collective bargaining. Traditionalists, in particular, also exhibited personal characteristics dissimilar from those of feminist respondents (See Figure 14).

The traditionalists were, for example, fundamentally different from the feminists in terms of age and education. Twenty-five percent of the traditionalists were born before World War II, compared with only eleven percent of the feminists. The majority of the traditionalists, seventy-five percent, held a hospital diploma as their highest degree. Traditionalists also worked fewer years and in different settings than feminist nurses. Seventy-five percent had spent most of their adult years as full-time homemakers, something none of the feminists had done. The other twenty-five percent worked primarily as hospital staff. One had some limited public health experience.[49] None, however, had worked in nursing education or administration, or as consultants and clinical specialists. Only one belonged to the ANA and she worked in an agency shop where membership in the local SNA was mandatory. This woman was also the only traditionalist who had joined a nursing specialty organization.[50]

In terms of family characteristics, traditionalists also differed markedly from feminists. The vast majority of traditionalists, seventy-five percent, had married only once. While twenty-five percent were either widowed or never married, none had experienced a divorce. They also tended to have larger families. Only 12.5 percent of the traditionalists were childless, compared to 28 percent of the feminists. More than three times as many of the traditionalists, 62.5 percent, had three to six children.

Not surprisingly traditionalists' values conflicted with those of feminists. Traditionalists, for example, believed men and women were inherently dissimilar. In their world view, the sexes performed complementary functions. As one explained, "Women and men are different. Each has different gifts, each can do some things the other can't."[51] Another agreed,

> I think men and women are very different. Their physical bodies are made differently and I think psychologically they are different also. I think they were made to complement each other.[52]

Traditionalists, therefore, totally supported the conventional, sexual division of labor. They believed "God originally intended woman to be wife of one husband and nurturer of children."[53] They also took for granted a divinely ordained, hierarchical social order in which males were dominant and females submissive. One woman explained her view of gender relationships in this way.

> I believe women should be submissive, so society can keep together. I revere my husband. Men have special abilities and wisdom that women don't have.[54]

Because they supported these conventional sex roles, traditionalists saw women's primary responsibility as the family. They disapproved of mothers' paid labor, arguing that a woman's first duty was to raise, supervise, and teach her children.[55] For traditionalists, women's employment was at best a marginal enterprise. Therefore they rejected the work place strategies adopted by feminist nurses. They perceived pay equity as an irrelevant and potentially harmful policy. One nurse argued that males should earn more than females because men supported families.[56] Traditionalists opposed unionization as a selfish and irresponsible strategy which harmed patients. As one traditionalist remarked,

> Collective bargaining is good only for attention-getting. I couldn't strike. I couldn't leave the patients. If a nurses' strike occurred locally, I would probably cross picket lines.[57]

Another woman, scandalized by an interview question about nurses' unions wrote, "That was *not* [italics hers] the way I was trained!"[58]

Traditionalists spurned the women's movement as an anti-family ideology. From their perspective the movement devalued the jobs women had performed well for generations. They perceived feminists as a self-centered, radical minority, riding roughshod over the lives of the basically satisfied majority.[59] A homemaker with two small children thus defined feminists as women "uncomfortable, insecure, or bitter about their own femininity and special role in society and the family."[60] Not surprisingly traditionalists vehemently opposed the Equal Rights Amendment. One characterized the feminist position on the ERA as "a fuss about nothing."[61] Another feared the Amendment would lead the government to draft women. Therefore she argued that the ERA "did more harm than good."[62] Traditionalist nurses, like women involved in the neo-conservative movement, felt uneasy about contemporary moral and family relationships. Although the

Amendment's effects were largely symbolic, they nevertheless saw it as an oppressive measure which would institutionalize "unnatural" gender roles.[63]

Traditionalists also opposed abortion, which they saw as "the ultimate selfish act."[64] From their perspective, feminists sanctioned reproductive choice because motherhood was inconvenient. As one nurse lamented, "Society is too concerned with taking the easy way out. People don't want to take responsibility."[65] All traditionalists believed a pregnant female should carry her child to term and relinquish it for adoption if she chose not to rear it herself. They acknowledged that this course of action presented hardships for the women involved. Nevertheless, they argued, it was the only responsible, moral option. One R.N. summarized the traditionalist position this way, "Life begins at conception, choice happens *before* [emphasis hers] conception. Women can practice abstinence or birth control."[66]

Feminists and traditionalists, then, held radically opposite opinions about the women's movement. Their views likewise represented extreme positions, different from those of perhaps the majority of nurses. The largest group within the Interview Subject Database, for example, held a mixture of feminist and traditionalist beliefs.

Middle-roaders' personal characteristics were also more varied than those of the other two groups (See Figure 14). They tended to be slightly younger than traditionalists, but older than feminists. Twenty-three percent had been born before World War II. They were also more highly educated than the traditionalists. Twelve (fifty-four percent) held a hospital diploma as their highest educational credential. Seven (thirty-two percent), however, had earned a BSN and three (fourteen percent) had a masters degree. Their length of employment ranged from two to thirty-one years, with the majority (forty-one percent) having worked in nursing for fifteen to twenty years. Their job experiences were more varied than those of either the feminists or traditionalists. Fifty-four percent had worked primarily in hospital general duty and twenty-three percent had worked as public health nurses, professional association officials, consultants, and clinical specialists. Another twenty-three percent were full-time homemakers. Fourteen (sixty-four percent) were ANA members and five (twenty-three percent) belonged to specialty organizations.

Middle-roaders likewise exhibited great diversity in their family characteristics. They were more likely to be married than feminists and more often divorced than traditionalists. Nineteen (eighty-six percent) were currently in their first marriage. Four percent had never married and ten percent were widowed or divorced. They had larger families than feminists, but fewer children than traditionalists. Two (ten percent) had no children and ten (forty-five percent) had one or two. Another forty-five percent had three to six children.

These middle-road nurses, many of whom had worked for a large portion of their lives, supported the feminist economic program. They advocated pay equity and collective bargaining. Predictably, those who belonged to the PNA were particularly vocal about nurses' right to organize.[67] Six (twenty-seven percent) were, in fact, local unit officers and another had organized nurses for the Association.[68] Three had been plaintiffs in pay equity lawsuits.[69] But those who were not unionized also acknowledged R.N.s' historically low wages and right to bargain collectively.[70] Some unorganized middle-roaders even sanctioned strikes, as long as employers maintained coverage for critically ill patients.[71]

Middle-road nurses upheld a woman's right to a career. They took pride in their own educational and professional achievements. One clinical specialist talked happily about her ten years of nursing and her intensive care certification.[72] An operating room nurse also spoke enthusiastically of her work and professional memberships.[73] A third woman — with expertise in cardiac care, surgical nursing, pediatrics, and rehabilitation — took pride in the fact that "I could financially support myself from graduation onward."[74] A number of middle-roaders left nursing or worked part-time during their children's pre-school years. As one said, "You have to re-prioritize after you have children."[75] But even those who had temporarily left paid labor asserted their right to return to nursing.[76]

Along with acknowledging women's rights to careers, middle-roaders argued the need for a more egalitarian family structure. They wanted husbands to perform domestic chores and care for children, particularly in families where wives worked outside the home. A hospital staff nurse explained,

> I believe in sharing household responsibilities. My mother-in-law worked outside the home so my husband can do everything. I don't like macho attitudes. And there are no more "Leave-it-to-Beaver" moms.[77]

Nor did middle-roaders believe that husbands should unilaterally control the family, as traditionalists did. One woman expressed the following views about marriage.

> In Genesis I the Bible says God made Adam's rib into Eve, not Adam's foot. I willingly *let* [italics mine] my husband be head of the household. But I'm not going to roll over for my husband either.[78]

At the same time, however, middle-road nurses embraced a number of traditional attitudes about gender. They believed women *were* fundamentally different from men. As one remarked,

> Women are not physically equal to men, although intellectually they are [equal]. But they're not identical. Otherwise, what's the point in having two sexes?[79]

Middle-roaders also saw women as innately more nurturing than men. They agreed, therefore, with traditionalists that females should bear primary responsibility for child-rearing. One mother of two explained, "People in the United States don't take care of their children anymore. *Mothers* [emphasis mine] need to be accountable for their children."[80] Another middle-roader believed women should choose careers compatible with motherhood. Referring to the mobilization of females during the Persian Gulf War, she argued that "The military is not for single women with children to raise."[81]

Middle-road nurses expressed a diversity of opinions about abortion. Only three (fourteen percent) defined themselves as pro-choice.[82] Four (eighteen percent) displayed ambivalence about the issue. They found abortion personally repugnant and morally unacceptable. Yet they reluctantly believed it should be legal for constitutional reasons. They also recognized that, in some circumstances, pregnancy endangered a woman's life. One middle-roader, who had briefly worked in obstetrics, was "bothered by abortion." But she also believed "women had the right to privacy and choice."[83] A public health nurse explained her position in this way.

> I believe women have many choices in prevention of pregnancy. I do not support abortion for moral and health reasons. Abortion is not a personal option, *but I don't tell others what to do* [italics mine].[84]

Fifteen (sixty-eight percent) middle-road nurses, however, vehemently opposed legalized abortion. They shared traditionalists' views about fetal life and the importance of motherhood. But middle-roaders also expressed concern about the impact of abortion on women themselves. They fretted about physical complications and post-abortion syndrome.[85] They feared easy access to abortion would lessen public support for government programs to aid poor women and children. One middle-road nurse explained,

> Intelligent women with career goals shouldn't feel as though they *have* [emphasis hers] to support abortion. They should push for services for pregnant women instead.[86]

Middle-roaders also rejected the Equal Rights Amendment, but for different reasons than traditionalists. For one thing, they perceived it as irrelevant. A hospital staff nurse and union activist accurately summarized this position when she commented, "I think the ERA is overrated."[87] A retired SNA official further suggested that comparable worth legislation would be more helpful to nurses than vague constitutional guarantees of equality.[88] Middle-roaders doubted whether the government could, in fact, guarantee equal treatment. As one explained,

> I don't have a problem *per se* [emphasis hers] with ERA, but I don't see a need for it. You fight sexual prejudice on a one-by-one basis. Attitudes only change slowly.[89]

Several middle-roaders also expressed concern that the ERA might actually hurt women. They feared constitutional equality would propel military women into combat, or jeopardize mothers' rights to child support.[90] Abortion opponents disliked the ERA because they saw a linkage between the two issues.[91]

Finally, despite their approval for the women's movement's economic platform, middle-roaders did not define themselves as feminists. Middle-road nurses tended to associate the movement with the negative stereotypes discussed above. For example two of the PNA 1986 strike leaders, who supported reproductive choice and comparable worth, viewed feminists as radical and militant. They explained,

> We don't get bent out of shape about women's problems. We don't march... The doctors call me a "women's libber," but I'm not.[92]

A public health nurse, who had filed a sex discrimination suit in 1974, had similar perceptions. She therefore took great pains to distinguish herself from feminists.

> I didn't read books or go to rallies. I didn't march. I didn't burn my bra.[93]

Middle-roaders also complained that the women's movement was still insensitive to females who had chosen traditional, feminine roles. A homemaker with three young children, for example, complained that feminists treated her "like my brain had deteriorated."[94] Other middle-road nurses rejected feminism because of its connection with the ERA and reproductive choice. Two R.N.s, who were very sympathetic to the movement's economic platform, opposed women's liberation for exactly these reasons.

> I'm a feminist at heart, but I'm not aligned with the feminist movement. They don't represent American women. I don't like the connection with abortion.[95]

> I'm not a feminist by current definition, but I believe in equality. Feminists wouldn't want me. They only want members who are pro-coice and pro-ERA. Those are their most important agenda items.[96]

Middle-road nurses, then, held a mixture of feminist and traditionalist beliefs. They supported the women's movement's economic program. But they did not entirely reject the sexual division of labor, nor were they in complete agreement with feminists about the ERA or abortion. Like their more traditional colleagues, middle-roaders perceived feminists as militant, out-of -the-mainstream radicals.

It is not completely clear whether life circumstances influenced these nurses' values or whether beliefs about gender determined career and family decisions. What is clear is that strong linkages existed between education, work experience, professional memberships, family status, and beliefs about sex roles. To some extent age also influenced women's attitudes (See Figure 14).

Traditionalist nurses' lives closely followed the patterns of earlier generations of women. One-quarter of the interview sample had been born and, in some cases, trained in hospital schools prior to World War II. Even those born later generally received their professional education through apprenticeship programs. Traditionalists rarely enrolled in college, either as new high school graduates or as already licensed nurses. Regardless of their age cohort, they tended to work rather briefly as hospital staff, then leave paid labor for full-time homemaking. If they resumed nursing it was only after their children were older and their domestic responsibilities somewhat lighter. They did not belong to professional organizations. Since they had lived rather conventional lives, they did not feel constrained by societal expectations of women. Traditionalists, therefore, did not express a need for personal liberation. Furthermore, they couldn't understand why their feminist colleagues were making such a fuss. They disapproved of the women's movement because they believed it devalued their own choices and lifestyles.

Middle-road R.N.s were, as a group, slightly younger than traditionalists. They were also more likely to possess a BSN and belong to professional associations. Although the majority worked as general duty staff, a sizable number of the sample held jobs as clinical specialists or in fields outside the hospital. Twenty-three percent were homemakers who planned to someday return to nursing. Middle-roaders worked outside the home for extended periods, often combining employment with motherhood. Like traditionalists, they lived primarily in nuclear families. They identified with feminism's economic platform, yet rejected other aspects of the movement.

Feminist nurses, on the other hand, were well-educated women, worked in autonomous and prestigious jobs, and belonged to professional organizations. Eighty-nine percent of the sample possessed at least a masters degree and ninety-five percent worked in fields such as nursing education, administration, and public health. All had been active in the ANA. None were full-time homemakers. These nurses were more likely than either traditionalists or middle-roaders to live outside the nuclear family. As primary earners and professionals they had faced the sex hierarchy and gender discrimination. As baby boomers they were also influenced by the social upheaval of the 1960s. They wanted, therefore, to free women from tradition and foster female independence.

Most rank-and-file R.N.s, however, did not possess the same characteristics as the feminist elite during the 1970s and early 1980s. In terms of education and occupation, American nurses most closely resembled middle-roaders. Despite the growth of higher education, only twenty-five and thirty percent of employed nurses held college degrees in 1980 and 1983.[97] Between 1977 and 1980 one-half to two-thirds of nurses worked as hospital staff. Only fifteen to nineteen percent held positions in administration or education. Slightly more than one percent were nurse-practitioners.[98] In other ways the rank-and-file mirrored the traditionalist sample. Women born before World War II comprised 28.6 percent of employed nurses in 1980.[99] Only thirteen to twenty percent belonged to the ANA during the late 1970s and early 1980s. Considerably fewer, 1.5 to 2.0 percent, held NLN membership.[100]

Understanding the differences among R.N.s explains why the relationship between nursing and the women's movement was fraught with obstacles. Hospital-educated, general duty staff — still the majority of nurses in the late 1970s and early 1980s — rejected feminism because they perceived it as denigrating their own lives. These women were comfortable with the conventional, nurturing roles of wife, mother, and care-giver. They saw feminists as selfish, immoral, anti-family, unfeminine radicals bent on destroying American society. Many nurses believed that "women's libbers," with their interest in male-dominated professions, felt only contempt for women in feminized jobs. Even some nursing activists, like the middle-roaders involved in the PNA, expressed ambivalence about supporting feminist groups such as NOW.

This hostility and ambivalence divided the profession, thereby limiting what feminist nurses could potentially accomplish. It also explains such phenomena as the conservative backlash against women's liberation during the 1980s.

The women's movement, however, did influence nursing. Feminism legitimized certain types of grievances and tactics, at least for college-educated, continuously employed baby boomers. Many of these women denied that they were feminists. At the same time, though, they defended their right to a career, called for a more egalitarian family structure, and embraced pay equity and collective bargaining. Thus while they rejected the feminist label, they accepted many of the movement's tenets. Nurse-activists did have many disappointments during the 1970s and early 1980s. They failed, for example, to institutionalize comparable worth or stop M.D.s' opposition to expanded roles. Yet, because of the way in which the women's movement affected younger R.N.s' attitudes, feminist nurses could claim some successes along with their losses.

Endnotes

1. Ashley, "Nursing and Early Feminism," 1467.

2. Blum, *Between Feminism and Labor,* 25; Goldfield, *The Decline of Organized Labor in the United States,* 103, 166-172; Hewlitt, *A Lesser Life,* 119, 132, 280, 353-354; "Partial Report of the Human Rights Committee," *AFSCME 25th Convention,* 68-70.

3. Blum, *Between Feminism and Labor,* 52.

4. Faye D. Ginsburg, *Contested Lives: The Abortion Debate in an American Community* (Berkeley: University of California Press, 1989), 43-54; Hewlitt, *A Lesser Life,* 197-211; Klatch, *Women of the New Right,* 5; Luker, *Abortion and the Politics of Motherhood,* 126-157; Mansbridge, *Why We Lost the ERA,* 3-7, 90-117, 174-177.

5. Elizabeth Harding, "Letters," *Nursing Outlook* 23 (May 1975): 284.

6. Kritek and Glass, "Nursing: A Feminist Perspective," 182.

7. Sharon A. Penny-Hopkins, "Moving into *The Second Stage:* An Interview with Betty Friedan," *Nursing Outlook* 29 (November 1981): 666.

8. Penny-Hopkins, "Moving into *The Second Stage,*" 666-667.

9. Susan W. Talbott and Connie N. Vance, "Involving Nursing in a Feminist Group - NOW," *Nursing Outlook* 29 (October 1981): 595.

10. Connie Vance, et al., "An Uneasy Alliance: Nursing And The Women's Movement," *Nursing Outlook* 33 (November/December 1985): 281.

11. Amenta, "Nurses NOW," 2; Subject #12; Beverly A. Trax, "Nurses' NOW: A History," Special Collections, Hillman Library, University of Pittsburgh, 2.

12. Subject #5.

13. Richard F. Newcomb, "Memo From The Editor," *RN* 35 (April 1972): 9.

14. "Nurses N.O.W.," *RN* 41 (April 1978): 13; Patricia Rogers, "How sexism haunts nursing," *RN* 42 (February 1979): 105.

15. "Nurses Notebook," *Nursing 73* 3 (May 1973): 50.

16. "Profile," *Nursing 74* 4 (April 1974): 8.

17. Hewlitt, *A Lesser Life*, 185-186; Mansbridge, *Why We Lost the ERA*, 103.

18. In 1972 when *RN* boasted a circulation of 250,000 the ANA and NLN had 166,676 and 14,130 nurse members respectively. Similarly during its first decade of publication, *Nursing* had 526,000 subscribers compared to the 161,188 nurses who belonged to the ANA. See "A Message From the Publisher," *RN* 36 (June 1973): 7; ANA, *Facts, '72-'73*, 64, 68; ANA, *Facts, '82-'83*, 117; Daniel L. Cheyney, "Publisher's Memo," *Nursing 81* 11 (January 1981): 5.

19. Subjects #1, #2, #3, and #26.

20. Subject #8.

21. Subject #9.

22. "ANA President Goes to White House," *AJN* 76 (August 1976): 1220; "ERA Supporters Work Against Clock as Deadline Looms," *AJN* 82 (February 1982): 212; "House Tackles Pay Equity Issue; Kennedy to Introduce Legislation," *AJN* 83 (January 1983): 7, 32.

23. For a discussion of autonomy within nursing education, public health, and administration see Melosh, *"The Physician's Hand,"* 126-128; Reverby, *Ordered to Care*, 70, 110; Tomes, " 'Little World of Our Own,' " 469-472.

24. Cleland, "Sex Discrimination," 1546-1547.

25. Thetis Group and Joan Roberts, "Exorcising The Ghosts of The Crimea," *Nursing Outlook* 22 (June 1974): 369-370; Penny A. McCarthy, "Will Faculty Practice Make Perfect?" *Nursing Outlook* 29 (March 1981): 163; Joan T. Roberts and Thetis M. Group, "The Women's Movement and Nursing," *Nursing Forum* 11, no. 3 (1973): 320-321.

26. Sharon C. Bridgwater, "Organizational Autonomy for Nursing Education," *Journal of Nursing Education* 18 (January 1979): 5-7; Edelstein, "Equal Rights for Women," 297; McBride, "A Married Feminist," 754-755.

27. Edith P. Lewis, "The Devil Within," *Nursing Outlook* 22 (June 1974): 367.

28. Rosella Schlotfeldt, "Reaction," *AJN* 72 (August 1972): 1449.

29. McBride, "A Married Feminist," 756.

30. Denise Benton Webster, "A Study of How Women Are Reflected in Nursing Text-books Used To Teach Obstetrics-Gynecology," *Nursing Forum* 16, no. 3 and 4 (1977): 289.

31. Bullough and Bullough, "Sex Discrimination in Health Care," 43; Diane H. Ross, "Letters," *AJN* 78 (February 1978): 217; Subject #8.

32. This analysis is based on personal and telephone interviews, conducted by the author, with feminist, traditionalists and middle-road nurses. These interviews occurred between June 1989 and April 1991 and will henceforth be referred to as the Interview Subject Database. Subjects were identified through both snowball interviewing techniques and organizational literature. A copy of the questionnaire is included in Appendix 2.

33. Subject #20.

34. Subjects #1, #3, #4, #12, #17, #19, and #25.

35. Subjects #8 and #22.

36. Subjects #2, #5, #6, #9, #11, #18, #23, and #24.

37. Subjects #5, #11, #19, #23, #24, and #25.

38. Subjects #8, #9, #12, and #25.

39. Subject #22.

40. Subjects #1, #2, and #3.

41. Subjects #8, #9, #12, and #25.

42. Subject #6.

43. Subject #20.

44. Subjects #1, #2, #5, #6, and #17.

45. Subject #6.

46. Subjects #2 and #5.

47. Subject #20.

48. Subject #8.

49. Subject #45, interview by author, mail questionnaire, 16 April 1991.

50. Subject #38, interview by author, 21 March 1991, Harrisburg, Pennsylvania.

51. Subject #44, interview by author, 15 April 1991, Lebanon, Pennsylvania.

52. Subject #45.

53. Subject #46, interview by author, mail questionnaire, 17 April 1991.

54. Subject #28, interview by author, tape recording, 28 February 1991, Marysville, Pennsylvania.

55. Subjects #38, #44, #46.

56. Subject #38.

57. Subject #44.

58. Subject #30, interview by author, mail questionnaire, 4 March 1991.

59. Subject #27, interview by author, 19 February 1991, Harrisburg, Pennsylvania; Subject #28 and #38.

60. Subject #46.

61. Subject #44.

62. Subject #27.

63. Chalmers, *And the Crooked Places Made Straight*, 165; Mansbridge, *Why We Lost the ERA*, 37-43.

64. Klatch, *Women of the New Right*, 129.

65. Subject #27.

66. Subject #44.

67. Subject #7; Subject #10; Subject #13; Subject #14; Subject #15; Subject #16; Subject #21, interview by author, telephone, 6 September 1989; Subject #29, interview by author, tape recording, 4 March 1991, Harrisburg, Pennsylvania; Subject #31, interview by author, 7 March, 1991, Harrisburg, Pennsylvania; Subject #36, interview by author, 18 March 1991, Camp Hill, Pennsylvania; Subject #37, interview by author, 20 March 1991, Hummelstown, Pennsylvania; Subject #39, interview by author, 22 March 1991, Harrisburg, Pennsylvania; Subject #42, interview by author, 9 April 1991, Annville, Pennsylvania; Subject #47, interview by author, 21 April 1991, Harrisburg, Pennsylvania.

68. Subjects #7, #10, #13, #14, #15, #16, and #21.

69. Subjects #13, #14, and #15.

70. Subject #32, interview by author, tape recording, 7 March 1991, Harrisburg, Pennsylvania; Subject #33, interview by author, 12 March 1991, Dillsburg, Pennsylvania.

71. Subject #36; Subject #43, interview by author, 11 April 1991, Hershey, Pennsylvania.

72. Subject #36.

73. Subject #32.

74. Subject #43.

75. Subject #36.

76. Subjects #32 and #36; Subject #41, interview by author , 9 April 1991, Hershey, Pennsylvania.

77. Subject #47.

78. Subject #29.

79. Subject #33.

80. Subject #29.

81. Subject #33.

82. Subjects #13, #14, and 16.

83. Subject #7.

84. Subject #10.

85. Subject #34, interview by author, 14 March 1991, Carlisle, Pennsylvania; Subjects #31, #33, #36, and #37.

86. Subject #35, interview by author, 15 March 1991, Hershey, Pennsylvania.

87. Subject #21.

88. Subject #7.

89. Subject #43.

90. Subjects #35, #37, and #47.

91. Subjects #34 and #36; Subject #48, interview by author , 30 April 1991, Dillsburg, Pennsylvania.

92. Subjects #13 and #14.

93. Subject #15.

94. Subject #41.

95. Subject #35.

96. Subject #43.

97. ANA, *Facts, '80-'81*, 6; ANA, *Facts About Nursing, 84-85* (New York: ANA, 1985), 18.

98. ANA, *Facts, '80-'81*, 10; ANA, *Facts, '82-'83*, 9.

99. ANA, *Facts, '82-'83*, 10.

100. ANA, *Facts, '72-'73*, 64, 68; ANA, *Facts, '76-'77*, 73, 79; ANA, *Facts, '82-'83*, 115, 117; ANA, *Facts, 84-85*, 112.

Conclusion

During the late 1960s, 1970s, and 1980s feminist nurses of every strand asked questions. In college classrooms, health care agencies, convention halls, and courtrooms they questioned the gender hierarchy. They also devised tactics which attempted, with mixed results, to combat this sexism. These strategies spoke to their experiences as workers in a woman's field. At the same time traditionalist and middle-of-the-road nurses questioned feminism's philosophy, agenda, and relevance.

This study has raised and answered a number of questions about nurses' experiences during these years. Specifically it has addressed the issues of why certain groups of nurses came to identify strongly with their work roles, and how such women regarded the re-emerging feminist movement. It has also analyzed how R.N.s used feminist rhetoric and tactics to attack work place problems. Finally, it has examined why other nurses found the women's movement threatening and distasteful.

After World War II, as the transformation of American health care fueled a massive demand for workers and employers made accommodations, married R.N.s re-entered the work force. These women often behaved as supplemental wage earners, whose salaries helped solidify their families' middle class status. Some portrayed themselves, at least publicly, as altruistic professionals sacrificing domesticity in the face of the personnel shortage. While married women's employment alone did not change beliefs about gender, it did restructure nursing into a work force of wives and mothers. Married women's employment also provided the next generation of R.N.s with important role models. It was these baby boomers — increasingly likely to be college educated and career committed — along with an older group of elite nurses, who identified strongly with both their profession and the women's movement.

These college-educated, often young R.N.s, with prestigious and autonomous jobs, became disgusted with the sexism within the health care system. As primary earners and professionals they expected, but did not receive, salaries and status commensurate with their self-images. Their frustration coincided with the reemergence of feminism.

Nurses learned about the women's movement from a variety of sources. Universities, the professional associations, the national media, friends, teachers, and colleagues played a role in the process of consciousness-raising. While feminist nurses all agreed that gender was socially constructed and that women should fight for equality with men, they supported different strands of the movement. Liberal feminists, like those of Nurses NOW, focused on gaining parity with male medical professionals. Radical feminists, such as the nurses of Cassandra, seemed more interested in completely overturning a patriarchal health care system and society.

Feminist nurses, however, generally agreed that R.N.s were entitled to higher salaries, more autonomy, and respect from male physicians and administrators. Consequently nursing engaged in litigation, embraced the pay equity movement, and developed new practice models. Roughly one-quarter of nurses unionized and negotiated for both better compensation and for issues of concern to female workers — maternity leave, pregnancy disability, and part-time benefits. Other R.N.s, disgusted with stagnant salaries, poor working conditions, and unappreciative physicians left the profession.

Feminist nurses, however, met with limited success. Several of the tactics mentioned above carried professional risks. Work place problems became more difficult to resolve in the conservative political and unstable economic climates of the 1980s. Nurses sometimes met with rejection from the larger women's movement. They also encountered scorn in certain segments of the professional media.

Moreover, feminists never convinced the majority of nurses to adopt their perspective or to ally themselves with the women's movement. This was due, in large part, to the fact that the feminist minority had very different personal characteristics and life experiences than those of the rank-and-file. Traditionalist nurses, for example, were more often born before World War II, educated in apprenticeship programs, and employed in hospitals. They saw the women's movement, and the nursing elite who supported it, as threatening forces. From the traditionalists' perspective feminism undermined the roles of wife, mother and caregiver. It both devalued their lifestyles and encouraged women to be selfish. Traditionalists saw no need for a women's movement because they wholeheartedly supported more conventional and conservative notions about gender.

Feminists and traditionalists represented opposite poles of the issue. A third group of nurses expressed ambivalence about the women's movement. These middle-roaders were generally baby boomers, career-minded, and often highly educated. They accepted the need for comparable worth and equal opportunity. Workers, as well as wives and mothers, they wanted an equitable division of labor within the home. Yet they did not completely reject convention gender roles. They also did not see themselves as feminists and often failed to support such policies as ERA ratification and reproductive choice.

The experiences of feminist nurses parallelled those of countless other female workers in the years after World War II. Smaller family size, the expansion of the clerical and service sectors, dropping of the marriage bar, and the desire for a middle class lifestyle propelled older, married women into the paid labor force during the 1950s and 1960s. By the 1970s younger females joined them. Inflation drove some of these baby boomers to seek employment. Others, primarily the ever-growing, college-educated segment, worked for intellectual stimulation and personal satisfaction. These younger women, along with a cadre of older and continuously employed female workers, saw themselves as professionals and primary earners. They therefore demanded equitable salaries and opportunities. They also felt frustrated by the discrimination they encountered.[1]

These disillusioned female workers discovered a re-emerging women's movement. At the same time experiences with civil rights and student organizations gave younger women a philosophy and set of tactics useful in dealing with gender discrimination. During the1960s, while older professional women lobbied for the Equal Pay Act and Title VII, younger feminists challenged patriarchal family arrangements. By the 1970s the two strands merged somewhat. Liberal feminist organizations such as NOW, for example, championed reproductive choice while radicals supported the ERA.[2] Many of these early feminists, like lawyers Mary Eastwood and Pauli Murray, worked in male-dominated professions.[3] Working daily with men, dealing with discrimination, watching less competent males succeed made these women particularly sensitve to gender inequality.[4] But, as this study has shown, women in the historically female occupations — particularly those who were young, highly educated, and employed in prestigious jobs — also identifed with feminism.

This re-emergence of the women's movement and its impact on American females constituted one of the major social phenomenon of the post-World War II period. Nowhere has this been more evident than in the lives of women born after the war. In some ways baby boomers returned to the marriage and fertility patterns established earlier in the twentieth century. They married at later ages than their parents, bore fewer children, and were more likely to divorce.[5] But in other ways these younger women were a unique generation. Between 1966 and 1984 they both doubled their college attendance and increasingly enrolled in previously male-dominated professional schools. By the mid-1980s females composed one-third of the entrants in law, medical, architecture, and business programs. They also exhibited new employment patterns. The working mothers of the 1950s and early 1960s were primarily the parents of school-aged children.[6] By 1980, however, forty-five percent of mothers of preschoolers were employed, a dramatic increase from the 11.9 percent who worked outside the home in 1950.[7] Attitudes changed along with behavior. During the late 1970s and early 1980s baby boomers expressed "almost universal approval" of mothers' paid labor.[8] Similarly, by 1980 college-going women exhibited as much career orientation as their male classmates.[9]

At the same time that feminism influenced younger women's choices, it divided the American people. Fears about mothers in combat, unisex public toilets, and the potential end of child support led traditionalists to bitterly and successfully oppose the ERA.[10] More than twenty years after *Roe v. Wade*, abortion is still a hotly contested political issue. Conservatives lament the loss of family values and blame feminists for such problems as crime and teenage pregnancy. They argue that the women's movement creates these difficulties by promoting female self-interest at the expense of the family.[11] Even some younger, employed women, such as the middle-road nurses in the Interview Subject Database, expressed discomfort with the feminist label. Both the American media and right-wing conservatives, who have portrayed "women's libbers" as strident and man-hating lesbians, bear some responsibility for these negative impressions. But the "guerrilla theater" tactics of some radical feminists and the "Why a Nurse Not a Doctor?" mentality also alienated some potential supporters.

Americans will argue over women's equality for some years to come. As conservative politicans continue to win office, debate over public policy matters, like abortion rights, reach a new intensity. Issues such as affirmative action and sexual harassment also create bitter controversy. Questions raised by the women's movement in the 1960s, 1970s, and 1980s have still not been resolved. All Americans — feminists, traditionalists, and middle-roaders — must work together to find the answers.

Endnotes

1. Cherlin, *Marriage, Divorce, Remarriage*, 50-52; Evans, *Personal Politics*, 15-21; Goldin, *Understanding the Gender Gap*, 174-176; May, *Homeward Bound*, 162-168, 209-219.

2. Evans, *Personal Politics*, 18-23, 199-217, 231.

3. Evans, *Personal Politics*, 19.

4. Kessler-Harris, *Out to Work*, 308-310.

5. Cherlin, *Marriage, Divorce, Remarriage*, 7-10, 21-23; May, *Homeward Bound*, 39-40, 221; McLaughlin et al., *Changing Lives*, 56-61, 126-129.

6. Cherlin, *Marriage, Divorce, Remarriage*, 51; Crispell, "Myths of the 1950s," 42; McLaughlin et al., *Changing Lives*, 32-39, 95.

7. Cherlin, *Marriage, Divorce, Remarriage*, 50-51; McLaughlin et al., *Changing Lives*, 32-34, 93-95.

8. McLaughlin et al., *Changing Lives*, 180-181.

9. Hillman, "The Effects Of College Going," 101-104; McLaughlin et al., *Changing Lives*, 175-176.

10. Klatch, *Women of the New Right*, 131-139; Mansbridge, *Why We Lost the ERA*, 90-117.

11. Klatch, *Women of the New Right*, 120-121.

APPENDIX 1:

Feminist Nursing Leaders, 1970-1986

The following appendix includes each nurse's highest educational credential, pertinent work experiences, professional and feminist association memberships, and areas of specialization between 1970 and 1986. Places of employment are listed chronologically from early to most recent. Sources are cited in the Bibliography.

JoAnn Ashley – Ed.D.; Assistant Professor at Pennsylvania State University, Associate Professor at Northern Illinois University; National Organization of Women; Nursing education, History of nursing

Bonnie Bullough – Ph.D.; Professor at California State University, Dean of Nursing at the State University of New York-Buffalo; American Nurses Association, Fellow of the American Academy of Nursing; History of nursing

Teresa Christy – Ed.D.; Professor at the University of Iowa; American Nurses Association, Fellow of the American Academy of Nursing, National Organization of Women; Nursing education, History of nursing

Virginia Cleland – Ph.D.; Professor at Wayne State University; American Nurses Association, Fellow of the American Academy of Nursing, Women's Equity Action League; Sociology

Eunice Cole – B.S.N.; Self-employed home health care consultant; American Nurses Association, Nurses Coalition for Action in Politics; Hospital staff and office nursing

Donna Diers – M.S.N.; Dean of Nursing at Yale University; Fellow of the American Academy of Nursing, Sigma Theta Tau (honorary nursing sorority); Psychiatric nursing

Claire Fagin – Ph.D.; Department Chair at the City University of New York, Dean of Nursing at the University of Pennsylvania; American Nurses Association, Fellow of the American Academy of Nursing, National League for Nursing; Mental health, Nurse-practitioners

Jeanne Fonesca – M.S.N.; Associate editor of *Nursing Outlook;* New York State Nurses Association, National League for Nursing; Nursing education, Public health

Ada Jacox – Ph.D.; Professor at the University of Iowa; American Nurses Association; Collective bargaining, Psychiatric nursing

Edith Patton Lewis – M.S.N.; Editor of *Nursing Outlook;* American Nurses Association, National League for Nursing; Journalism, psychiatric nursing

Mary Mallison – B.S.N.; Editor of the *American Journal of Nursing;* Georgia Nurses Association; Hospital staff nursing, Public health

Angela McBride – Ph.D.; Assistant Professor at Yale University, Associate Dean of Nursing at Indiana University; American Nurses Association, Fellow of the American Academy of Nursing; Psychiatric nursing

Penny McCarthy – M.S.N.; Editor of *Nursing Outlook;* American Nurses Association, National League for Nursing, National Organization for Women; Nursing education, Psychiatric nursing

Barbara Nichols – M.S.N.; Director of Nursing at St. Vincent's Hospital (Milwaukee), California Nurses Association; American Nurses Association, Fellow of the American Academy of Nursing; Hospital staff development

Thelma Schorr – B.S.N.; Editor of the *American Journal of Nursing;* American Nurses Association, National League for Nursing; Journalism, Hospital staff nursing

Barbara Schutt – M.S.N.; Editor of the *American Journal of Nursing;* American Nurses Association, Connecticut Nurses Association; Journalism, Collective bargaining

Rosella Schlottfeld – Ph.D.; Dean of Nursing at Case Western Reserve University; American Nurses Association, National League for Nursing; Nursing education, Nursing administration

Gloria Smith – Ph.D.; Dean of Nursing at the University of Oklahoma; American Nurses Association, Fellow of the American Academy of Nursing, Midwest Alliance of Nursing; Anthropology, Public health nursing

Margretta Styles – Ed.D.; Dean of Nursing at Wayne State University, Dean of Nursing at the University of California – San Francisco; American Nurses Association, Midwest Alliance of Nursing; Nursing education, Pay equity

Anne Zimmerman – B.S.N.; Director of the Illinois Nurses Association; American Nurses Association; Collective bargaining

Activist Nurses' Questionnaire

Name _____

Year of Birth _____

Ethnic Background (Circle): Caucasian African-American Asian
Native American Other

Marital Status (Circle): Never Married Married Widowed
Divorced/Separated Cohabitating Remarried Other

Number of Children and Birthdates _____

Husband's Occupation (if applicable)_____

Father's Occupation _____

Mother's Occupation _____

Number of Brothers: Older_____ Younger_____

Number of Sisters: Older_____ Younger_____

Parents' Religious Affiliation (if applicable) _____

Your Current Religious Affiliation (if applicable) _____

Educational Background:

High School _____
Year Graduated_____
Location _____

Hospital Nursing School _____
Year Graduated_____
Location _____

Associate Degree Nursing Program _____
Year Graduated_____
Location _____

Bachelor of Nursing Program _____
Year Graduated_____
Location _____

Masters Program _____
Year Graduated_____
Location _____

Type of Degree _____

Other Relevant Educational Experiences (use back of sheet if necessary): _____
_____
_____
_____
_____
_____
_____

Work Experience:

First Job as a Nurse _____
Where _____
When _____
Briefly explain your responsibilities: _____
_____
_____
_____
_____
_____
_____
_____

Current Job _____
Where _____
How Long?_____   Title _____
Briefly explain your responsibilities: _____
_____
_____
_____
_____
_____
_____

What other jobs or professional experiences have you had as a nurse?
_____
_____
_____
_____
_____
_____
_____

What have been your greatest joys or achievements as a nurse?

_____

_____

_____

_____

_____

_____

_____

What have been your greatest frustrations or difficulties?

_____

_____

_____

_____

_____

_____

Professional Organizations:

List the names and dates of membership of any professional nursing organizations you have belonged to (use back of sheet if necessary).

_____

_____

_____

_____

_____

_____

_____

Offices Held:

_____

_____

_____

_____

_____

_____

_____

Committees or Special Projects:

_____
_____
_____
_____
_____
_____

Activist Experiences:

Your Primary Organization (Circle One):   Nurses NOW   Birthright
Pennsylvanians for Human Life   PNA Bargaining Unit

When did you first decide to join this organization? What factors influenced your decision? _____

_____
_____
_____
_____
_____
_____

When and where did you first participate in this organization?

_____
_____
_____
_____
_____
_____

Please describe the situation and how you participated.

_____
_____
_____
_____
_____
_____

Did you personally help establish any groups related to this organization? Which ones? Why did you establish these groups?

_____

_____

_____

_____

_____

_____

_____

Was your organization successful in achieving its goals? Why or why not? _____

_____

_____

_____

_____

_____

_____

Miscellaneous Questions:

Did you combine nursing with motherhood? If so, what special problems or frustrations did you encounter? _____

_____

_____

_____

_____

_____

Are you more or less satisfied with nursing than you were ten years ago? Why or why not? _____

_____

_____

_____

_____

_____

Nurses NOW, Birthright, and PHL members only: Have you had any experiences with unions — AFSCME, SEIU, 1199, etc.? A PNA or other state nurses association barganing unit? If so, please describe.

_____

_____

_____

_____

_____

_____

_____

Nurses NOW, Birthright, and PHL members only: Do you approve of collective bargaining for nurses? Why or why not?

_____

_____

_____

_____

_____

_____

Do you approve of the Equal Rights Amendment? Why or why not?

_____

_____

_____

_____

_____

_____

Do you approve of pay equity (comparable worth) for women workers? Have you actively worked to promote pay equity at your place of employment?_____

_____

_____

_____

_____

_____

_____

PNA Bargaining Unit and Nurses NOW members only: What is your position on abortion? _____

_____

_____

_____

_____

_____

_____

_____

Do you consider yourself a feminist? Why or why not? How would you define that term? _____

_____

_____

_____

_____

_____

_____

Do you know of any other nurses from your organization who would be willing to talk with me? If so, would you please give names and addresses (use back of sheet if necessary)? _____

_____

_____

_____

_____

_____

_____

Release Form:

Susan Rimby Leighow may use this questionnaire for such purposes as are necessary for writing her dissertation and subsequent publications.

_____   _____
(Signature)   (Date)

Bibliography

Nursing Articles, Publications, and Trade Journals

American Journal of Nursing. 33-86 (1933-1986).

American Nurses Association. *Convention Journal.* 1946-1972, 1982-1984.

_____. *Facts About Nursing, 1949-1987.* New York and Kansas City: American Nurses Association, 1949-1987.

Ashley, JoAnn. "Practice Oriented Theory." *Advances in Nursing Science* 1 (October 1978): 25.

_____. "Power in Structured Misogyny: Implications for the Politics of Care." *Advances in Nursing Science* 2 (April 1980): 3-22.

Bentivegna, Gail. "Labor Relations: Union Activity Increases Among Professionals." *Hospitals* 53 (April 1979): 131-139.

Bullough, Bonnie. "Legal Restrictions as a Barrier to Nurse Practitioner Role Development." *Pediatric Nursing* 10 (November/December 1984): 439-442.

Burgess, May Ayres. *Nurses, Patients, And Pocketbooks.* New York: Committee on the Grading of Nursing Schools, 1928.

Cassandra. *Cassandra: Radical Feminist Nurses Newsjournal* 1-5 (1982-1987).

Cleland, Virginia. "To End Sex Discrimination." *Nursing Clinics of North America* 9 (September 1974): 563-571.

Dock, Lavinia L. "Letters to the Editor." *American Journal of Nursing* 24 (July 1924): 834.

_____. "Some Urgent Social Claims." *American Journal of Nursing* 7 (April 1907): 895.

_____. "Letters to the Editor." *American Journal of Nursing* 8 (August 1908): 925-926.

Dustan, Laura C. "Characteristics of Students in Three Types of Nursing Education Programs," *Nursing Research* 13 (Spring 1964): 159-166.

Elliot, Clifton L. "Hospitals must face heavy unionization drives in '80s-part 1." *Hospitals* 55 (June 16, 1981): 55-58.

Fagin, Claire M., and Jill Glatter Nussbaum. "Parental Visiting Privileges in Pediatric Units." *Journal of Nursing Administration* 8 (March 1978): 24-27.

Fondiller, Shirley H. *The Entry Dilemma: The National League for Nursing and the Higher Education Movement, 1952-1972, With an Epilogue to 1983.* 2nd ed. New York: National League for Nursing, 1983.

Ford, Loretta C. "Physicians' Assistant: Why, Who, and How?" *AORN Journal* 15 (April 1972): 41-60.

Gortner, Susan. "Nursing Majors in Twelve Western Universities: A Comparison of Registered Nurse Students and Basic Senior Students." *Nursing Research* 17 (March-April 1968): 121-129.

Greenleaf, Nancy P. "Labor Force Participation among Registered Nurses and Women in Comparable Occupations." *Nursing Research* 32 (September/October 1983): 306-311.

Hughes, Everett C., Helen MacGill Hughes, and Irwin Deutscher. *Twenty Thousand Nurses Tell Their Story.* Philadelphia: J.B. Lippincott Company, 1958.

The Journal of Nursing Education. 1-24 (1962-1986).

Kaufman, Martin, ed. *Dictionary of American Nursing Biography.* New York: Greenwood Press, 1988.

Kohnke, Mary F., Ann Zimmern, and Jocelyn A. Greenidge. *Independent Nurse Practitioner.* Garden Grove, Ca.: Trainex Press, 1974.

Koncel, Jerome A. "Hospital Labor Relations Struggles Through Its Own Revolution." *Hospitals* 51 (April 1, 1977): 69-74.

Knopf, Lucille. *Registered Nurses Fifteen Years After Graduation.* New York: National League for Nursing, 1983.

"League Sees Change." *AORN Journal* 34 (July 1981): 98.

Metzger, Norman. "Hospital Labor Scene Marked by Union Issues." *Hospitals.* 54 (April 1980): 105-112.

Mitchell, Karen. "The Death of the Goose that Laid the Golden Egg." *Pediatric Nursing* 10 (March/April 1984): 101.

Miller, Michael H., and Lee Dodson. "Work Stoppage Among Nurses." *Journal of Nursing Administration* 6 (December 1976): 41-45.

Murray, Louisa M., and Donald R. Morris. "Professional Autonomy among Senior Nursing Students in Diploma, Associate Degree, and Baccalaureate Nursing Programs." *Nursing Research* 31 (September/October 1982): 311-313.

National League for Nursing. *NLN News.* 1951-1983.

National League for Nursing. "Nurse Career-Pattern Study: Baccalaureate Degree Nurses Ten Years After Graduation." *Hospital Topics* 57 (May/June 1979): 6.

Numeroff, Rita E., and Michael N. Abrams. "Collective bargaining among nurses: current issues and future prospects." *Health Care Management Review* 9 (Spring 1984): 61-67.

Nursing 3-16 (1973-1986).

Nursing Forum 1-24 (1962-1986).

Nursing Outlook 1-33 (1953-1986).

Oshin, Edith S. "How to Get Help For Your Education." *RN* 24 (November 1961): 44-51.

Patch, Frances B., and Stephanie Holaday. "Effects of Change in Professional Liability Insurance on Certified Nurse-Midwives." *Journal of Nurse-Midwifery* 34 (May/June 1989): 131-136.

The Pennsylvania Nurse 1-40 (1946-1986).

"Pennsylvania Takes COP to Court in Sex Discrimination Complaint." *Contact* 14 (December 1986): 1.

Pettengill, Marian Martin. "Multilateral Collective Barganing and the Health Care Industry: Implications for Nursing." *Journal of Professional Nursing* 1 (September-October 1985): 275-282.

Posluny, Susan M. "Feminist Friendship: Isabel Hampton Robb, Lavinia Lloyd Dock, and Mary Adelaide Nutting." *Image: Journal of Nursing Scholarship* 21 (Summer 1989): 64-70.

RN 35-49 (1972-1986).

Silver, Henry K., Loretta C. Ford, and Lewis R. Day. "The Pediatric Nurse-Practitioner Program." *The Journal of the American Medical Association* 204 (April 22, 1968): 298-302.

Webb, Christopher A. "The Nurse Today-'68." *RN* 31 (July 1968): 31-46.

Labor Union Periodicals

1199 News 10-21 (1975-1986).

Public Employee 44-47 (1979-1983).

Service Employee 34-42 (1975-1982).

Manuscript and Archival Collections

American Nurses Association. Convention Proceedings, 1946-1972. Mugar Library, Boston University.

National League for Nursing. Convention Proceedings, 1951-1983. National League for Nursing Headquarters, New York.

New York State School of Industrial and Labor Relations. Labor-Management Documentation Center Papers. The Martin P. Catherwood Library, Cornell University, Ithaca, New York.

Nurses NOW Papers. Special Collections, Hillman Library, University of Pittsburgh.

Pennsylvania Nurses Association. Collective Bargaining Papers. The Dorothy J. Novello Memorial Library, Pennsylvania Nurses Association Headquarters, Harrisburg, Pennsylvania.

Magazine and Newspaper Articles

Anderson, Harry, Erik P. Ipsen, and Rich Thomas. "Good News on the Economy." *Newsweek,* 29 June 1981, 55.

"As Prices Keep Spiraling-How People Are Tightening Their Belts." *U.S. News & World Report,* 24 December 1973, 15-20.

Clark, Matt. "Nurses: Few and Fatigued." *Newsweek,* 29 June 1987, 59-60.

Curran, Robert. "Strike Impending At 3 Regional State Hospitals." *The Tribune (Scranton, Pennsylvania)* , 19 January 1986, B1.

The Daily American (Somerset Pennsylvania), 23 January-1 February 1986.

"Inflation Grows Worse." *Time*, 27 March 1978, 58.

Killborn, Peter T. "Nurses get V.I.P. Treatment, Erasing Shortage." *New York Times*, 1 May 1990, 1.

Lewin, Tamar. "Women Are Becoming Equal Providers." *New York Times*, 11 May 1995, sec. 1.

"No Crash of '79 Coming Up." *Time*, 2 October 1978, 54-55.

"A Plan for Fighting the Double Digits." *Time*, 18 April 1977, 49-50.

Pennsylvania NOW, April 1974.

Pottsville (Pennsylvania) Republican, 22-30 January 1986.

Progress Notes (Nurses NOW), Fall 1977.

"Why All The Talk Of Recession." *U.S. News & World Report*, 24 December 1973, 11-12.

Government Documents

United States Department of Labor. *Impact of the 1974 Health Care Amendments to the NLRA on Collective Bargaining in the Health Care Industry*. Washington, D.C.: Government Printing Office, 1979.

Interviews

Edith Barnett. Interview by author. Tape recording, 26 February 1991. Washington, D.C.

Kathryn J. Grove. Interview by Alice M. Hoffman, *Kathryn J. Grove, Executive Director, 1968-1984, PNA Oral History Interviews, 1984-85*. Dorothy M. Novello Memorial Library. The Pennsylvania Nurses Association. Harrisburg, Pennsylvania.

Smith, Mary [pseud.]. Interview by author. Telephone, 27 February 1991. American Nurses Association Headquarters. Kansas City.

Subject #1. Interview by author. Telephone, 6 June 1989.

Subject #2. Interview by author. Tape recording, 7 June 1989. Pittsburgh, Pennsylvania.

Subject #3. Interview by author. Tape recording, 7 June 1989. Mars, Pennsylvania.

Subject #4. Interview by author. 8 June 1989. Pittsburgh, Pennsylvania.

Subject #5. Interview by author. 9 June 1989. Pittsburgh, Pennsylvania.

Subject #6. Interview by author. 9 June 1989. Pittsburgh, Pennsylvania.

Subject #7. Interview by author. 14 June 1989. Camp Hill, Pennsylvania.

Subject #8. Interview by author. Tape recording, 14 June 1989. Harrisburg, Pennsylvania.

Subject #9. Interview by author. 22 June 1989. Carbondale, Pennsylvania.

Subject #10. Interview by author. Tape recording, 23 June 1989. Mt. Carmel, Pennsylvania.

Subject #11. Interview by author. 23 June 1989. Norristown, Pennsylvania.

Subject #12. Interview by author. Telephone, 28 June 1989.

Subjects #13 and #14. Interview by author. Tape recording, 28 June 1989. Ashland, Pennsylvania.

Subject #15. Interview by author. Tape recording, 7 July 1989. Doylestown, Pennsylvania.

Subject #16. Interview by author. Tape recording, 13 July 1989. Harrisburg, Pennsylvania.

Subject #17. Interview by author. Tape recording, 20 July 1989. Harrisburg, Pennsylvania.

Subject #18. Interview by author. 26 July 1989. Hershey, Harrisburg, Pennsylvania.

Subject #19. Interview by author. 23 August 1989. Philadelphia, Pennsylvania.

Subject #20. Interview by author. Telephone, 28 August 1989.

Subject #21. Interview by author. Telephone, 29 September 1989.

Subject #22. Interview by author. Tape recording, 28 September 1989. Harrisburg, Pennsylvania.

Subject #23. Interview by author. Tape recording, 22 October 1989. Pittsburgh, Pennsylvania.

Subject #24. Interview by author. 23 October 1989. Monroeville, Pennsylvania.

Subject #25. Interview by author. Tape recording, 23 October 1989. Pittsburgh, Pennsylvania.

Subject #26. Interview by author. Tape recording, 24 October 1989. Pittsburgh, Pennsylvania.

Subject #27. Interview by author. 19 February 1991. Harrisburg, Pennsylvania.

Subject #28. Interview by author. Tape recording, 28 February 1991. Marysville, Pennsylvania.

Subject #29. Interview by author. Tape recording, 4 March 1991. Harrisburg, Pennsylvania.

Subject #30. Interview by author. Mail questionnaire. 4 March 1991.

Subject #31. Interview by author. 7 March 1991. Harrisburg, Pennsylvania.

Subject #32. Interview by author. Tape recording, 7 March 1991. Harrisburg, Pennsylvania.

Subject #33. Interview by author. 12 March 1991. Dillsburg, Pennsylvania.

Subject #34. Interview by author. 14 March 1991. Carlisle, Pennsylvania.

Subject #35. Interview by author. 15 March 1991. Hershey, Pennsylvania.

Subject #36. Interview by author. 18 March 1991. Camp Hill, Pennsylvania.

Subject #37. Interview by author. 20 March 1991. Hummelstown, Pennsylvania.

Subject #38. Interview by author. 21 March 1991. Harrisburg, Pennsylvania.

Subject #39. Interview by author. 22 March 1991. Harrisburg, Pennsylvania.

Subject #40. Interview by author. Mail questionnaire, 1 April 1991.

Subject #41. Interview by author. 9 April 1991. Hershey, Pennsylvania.

Subject #42. Interview by author. 9 April 1991. Annville, Pennsylvania.

Subject #43. Interview by author. 11 April 1991. Hershey, Pennsylvania.

Subject #44. Interview by author. 15 April 1991. Lebanon, Pennsylvania.

Subject #45. Interview by author. Mail questionnaire, 16 April 1991.

Subject #46. Interview by author. Mail questionnaire, 17 April 1991.

Subject #47. Interview by author. 21 April 1991. Harrisburg, Pennsylvania.

Subject #48. Interview by author. 30 April 1991. Dillsburg, Pennsylvania.

Subject #49. Interview by author. 2 May 1991. Harrisburg, Pennsylvania.

Books

Aaron, Benjamin, Joyce M. Najita, and James L. Stern, ed. *Public Sector Bargaining*. Washington, D.C.: The Bureau of National Affairs, Inc, 1988.

Ashley, JoAnn. *Hospitals, Paternalism, and the Role of the Nurse*. New York: Teachers College Press, 1976.

Blum, Linda. *Between Feminism and Labor: The Significance of the Comparable Worth Movement*. Berkeley: University of California Press, 1991.

Chalmers, David. *And the Crooked Places Made Straight: The Struggle for Social Change in the 1960s.* Baltimore: The Johns Hopkins University Press, 1991.

Cherlin, Andrew J. *Marriage, Divorce, Remarriage.* Cambridge, MA.: Harvard University Press, 1981.

Cott, Nancy F. *The Grounding of Modern Feminism.* New Haven: Yale University Press, 1987.

Dolan, Josephine A. *Nursing in Society: A Historical Perspective.* 14th ed. Philadelphia: W.B. Saunders Company, 1978.

Easterlin, Richard O. *Birth and Fortune: The Impact of Numbers on Personal Welfare.* New York: Basic Books, Inc., 1980.

Evans, Sara. *Born for Liberty: A History of Women in America.* New York: The Free Press, 1989.

_____. *Personal Politics: The Roots of Women's Liberation in the Civil Rights Movement and the New Left.* New York: Alfred A. Knopf, 1979.

Fink, Leon, and Brian Greenberg. *Upheaval in the Quiet Zone: A History of Hospital Workers Union, Local 1199.* Urbana: University of Illinois Press, 1989.

Gabin, Nancy F. *Feminism in the Labor Movement: Women and the United Auto Workers, 1935-1975.* Ithaca: Cornell University Press, 1990.

Garrison, Dee. *Apostles of Culture: The Public Librarian and American Society, 1875-1920.* New York: Macmillan, 1979.

Gilbert, James. *Another Chance: Postwar America, 1945-1968.* Philadelphia: Temple University Press, 1981.

Ginsburg, Faye D. *Contested Lives: The Abortion Debate in an American Community.* Berkeley: University of Califorina Press, 1989.

Gitlin, Todd. *The Sixties: Years of Hope, Days of Rage.* New York: Bantam Books, 1987.

Goldfield, Michael. *The Decline of Organized Labor in the United States.* Chicago: The University of Chicago Press, 1987.

Goldin, Claudia. *Understanding the Gender Gap.* New York: Oxford University Press, 1990.

Hartmann, Susan M. *The Home Front and Beyond: American Women in the 1940s*. Boston: Twayne Publishers, 1982.

Hewlitt, Sylvia Ann. *A Lesser Life: The Myth of Women's Liberation in America*. New York: Morrow and Company, Inc., 1986.

Hine, Darlene Clark. *Black Women in White: Racial Conflict and Cooperation in the Nursing Profession, 1890-1950*. Bloomington: Indiana University Press, 1989.

Jackson, Kenneth T. *Crabgrass Frontier: The Suburbanization of the United States*. New York: Oxford University Press, 1985.

Kalisch, Philip A., and Beatrice J. Kalisch. *The Advance of American Nursing*. 2nd ed. Boston: Little, Brown, and Company, 1986.

Kelley, Win, and Leslie Wilbur. *Teaching in The Community Junior College*. New York: Appleton-Century-Crofts, 1970.

Kessler-Harris, Alice. *Out to Work: A History of Wage-Earning Women in the United States*. New York: Oxford University Press, 1982.

Klatch, Rebecca E. *Women of the New Right*. Philadelphia: Temple University Press, 1987.

Klein, Ethel. *Gender Politics: From Consciousness to Mass Politics*. Cambridge, MA.: Harvard University Press, 1984.

Leavitt, Judith Walzer, ed. *Women and Health in America*. Madison: University of Wisconsin Press, 1984.

Lewin, David, Peter Feuille, and Thomas Kochan, ed. *Public Sector Labor Relations: Analysis and Readings*. New York: Thomas Horton & Daughters, 1977.

Litoff, Judy Barrett. *American Midwives: 1860 to the Present*. Westport, CT.: Greenwood Press, 1978.

Luker, Kristen. *Abortion and the Politics of Motherhood*. Berkeley: University of California Press, 1984.

Mansbridge, Jane J. *Why We Lost the ERA*. Chicago: University of Chicago Press, 1986.

May, Elaine Tyler. *Homeward Bound: American Families in the Cold War Era*. New York: Basic Books, Inc., 1988.

McLaughlin, Steven D., Barbara D. Melber, John O.G. Billy, Denise M. Zimmerle, Linda D. Winges, and Terry R. Johnson. *The Changing Lives of American Women.* Chapel Hill: The University of North Carolina Press, 1988.

Melosh, Barbara. *"The Physician's Hand:" Work Culture and American Nursing.* Philadelphia: Temple University Press, 1982.

Meyerowitz, Joanne, ed. *Not June Cleaver: Women and Gender in Postwar America, 1945-1960.* Philadelphia: Temple University Press, 1994.

Miller, James. *"Democracy is in the Streets:" From Port Huron to the Siege of Chicago.* New York: Simon and Schuster, 1987.

Reverby, Susan M. *Ordered to Care: The dilemma of American nursing, 1850-1945.* New York: Cambridge University Press, 1987.

Rix, Sara E., ed. *The American Woman 1988-89: A Status Report.* New York: W.W. Norton & Company, 1988.

Solomon, Barbara Miller. *In the Company of Educated Women: A History of Women and Higher Education in America.* New Haven: Yale University Press, 1985.

Starr, Paul. *The Social Transformation of American Medicine.* New York: Basic Books, Inc., 1982.

Stevens, Rosemary. *In Sickness and Wealth: American Hospitals in the Twentieth Century.* New York: Basic Books, Inc., 1989.

Ulrich, Laurel Thatcher. *Good Wives: Image and Reality in the Lives of Women in Northern New England, 1650-1750.* New York: Alfred A. Knopf, 1987.

Wechsler, Harold S. *The Qualified Student: A History of Selective College Admission in America.* New York: John Wiley & Sons, 1977.

Scholarly Articles

Brent, Nancy J. "The Nurse Practitioner After Sermchief and Fein: Smooth Sailing or Rough Waters?" *Valparaiso University Law Review* 21 (Winter 1987): 221-240.

Bullough, Bonnie. "The Current Phase In The Development of Nurse Practice Acts." *Saint Louis University Law Journal* 28, no. 2, (1984): 365-395.

Buhler-Wilkerson, Karen. "Caring in Its 'Proper Place:' Race and Benevolence in Charleston, South Carolina, 1813-1930." *Nursing Research* 41 (January/February 1992): 14-20.

_____. "Left Carrying the Bag: Experiments in Visiting Nursing, 1877-1909." *Nursing Research* 36 (January/February 1987): 42-47.

Cohn, Sara D. "Survey of Legislation on Third Party Reimbursement." *Law, Medicine, and Health Care* 11 (December 1983): 22-24.

Cott, Nancy F. "Feminist Theory and Feminist Movements: The Past Before Us," 49-62. In *What is Feminism?* edited by Juliet Mitchell and Ann Oakley. New York: Pantheon Books, 1986.

_____. "What's in a Name? The Limits of 'Social Feminism,' or Expanding the Vocabulary of Women's History." *Journal of American History* 76 (December 1989): 809-829.

Crispell, Diane. "Myths of the 1950s." *American Demographics* 14 (August 1992): 38-43.

Delaney, John Thomas. "Union Success in Hospital Representation Elections." *Industrial Relations* 20 (Spring 1981): 149-160.

Dowd, Nancy E. "The Metamorphosis of Comparable Worth." *Suffolk University Law Review* 20 (Winter 1986): 833-865.

Feldman, Roger, and Richard Scheffler. "The Union Impact on Hospital Wages and Fringe Benefits." *Industrial and Labor Relations Review* 35 (January 1982): 196-206.

Friss, Lois O'Brien. "Work Force Policy Perspectives: Registered Nurses." *Journal of Health Politics, Polity, and Law* 5 (Winter 1981): 696-719.

Goldin, Claudia. "The Meaning of College in The Lives of American Women: The Past One-Hundred Years." *National Bureau of Economic Research Working Paper Series* 4099 (June 1992).

Grimm, James W. "Women in Female-Dominated Professions." In *Women Working*, 293-315. edited by Ann H. Stromberg and Shirley Harkess. Palo Alto, CA.: Mayfield Publishing Co., 1978.

Gross, Edward. "Plus Ca Change...? The Sexual Structure of Occupations Over Time." *Social Problems* 16 (Fall 1968): 198-208.

Hirsch, Harold L., and John M. Studner. "The Nurse Practitioner (NP) in Action: Patients' Friend, Physicians' Foe?" *Medical Trial Technique Quarterly* (1985 annual): 37-76.

Kokklenberg, Edward C., and Donna R. Sockell. "Union Membership in the United States, 1973-1981." *Industrial and Labor Relations Review* 38 (July 1985): 497-543.

Kravitz, Diane. "Sexism In A Woman's Profession." *Social Work* 21 (November 1976): 421-426.

Lewin, David, and Shirley B. Goldenberg. "Public Sector Unionism in the U.S. and Canada." *Industrial Relations* 20 (Spring 1981): 239-254.

Lupica, Lois R. "Pay Equity-A 'Cockamaime' Idea? The Future of Health Care May Depend Upon It." *American Journal of Law and Medicine* 13, no. 4 (1988): 597-620.

Moskowitz, Seymour. "Pay Equity and American Nurses: A Legal Analysis." *St. Louis University Law Journal* 27 (November 1983): 801-854.

Peizer, Donna M. "A Social and Legal Analysis of the Independent Practice of Midwifery." *Berkeley Women's Law Journal* 2 (Fall 1986): 141-240.

Reverby, Susan M. "A Caring Dilemma: Womanhood and Nursing in Historical Perspective." *Nursing Research* 36 (January/February 1987): 5-11.

Seidman, Joel. "Nurses and Collective Bargaining." *Industrial and Labor Relations Review* 23 (April 1970): 335-351.

Spitzer, Walter O. "The Nurse Practitioner Revisited: Slow Death of a Good Idea." *The New England Journal of Medicine* 310 (April 9, 1984): 1049-1051.

Stelluto, George. "Earnings of Hospital Nurses, July 1966." *Monthly Labor Review* 90 (June 1967): 55-58.

Strober, Myra H., and Audri Gordon Lanford. "The Feminization of Public School Teaching: Cross-Sectional Analysis, 1850-1880." *Signs* 11 (Winter 1986): 212-235.

Tanimoto, Helene S., and Gail F. Inaba. "State employee bargaining: policy and organization. *Monthly Labor Review* 108 (April 1985): 51-55.

Tillery, Dale, and William L. Deegan. "The Evolution of Two-Year Colleges Through Four Generations." In *Renewing the American Community College,* edited by William L. Deegan, Dale Tillery, and Associates, 3-33. San Francisco: Jossey-Bass Publishers, 1985.

Wagner, David. "The Proletarianization of Nursing in the United States, 1932-1946." *International Journal of Health Services* 10, no. 2 (1980): 271-290.

Waite, Linda J. "Working Wives, 1940-1960." *American Sociological Review* 4 (February 1976): 65-80.

Weintraub, David. "A New Role for Nurses: The Nurse Practitioner." *Medical Trial Technique Quarterly* (1985 annual): 78-80.

Wriston, Sara. "Nurse Practitioner Reimbursement." *Journal of Health Politics, Policy, and Law* 6 (Fall 1981): 444-462.

Dissertations and Unpublished Papers

Armeny, Susan. "Resolute Enthusiasts: The Effort to Professionalize American Nursing, 1880-1915." Ph.D. diss., University of Missouri-Columbia, 1983.

Hillman, Sandra Mary. "The Effects of College Going Women's Current Values and Attitudes on the Decline in Enrollments to Baccalaureate Programs in Nursing." Ph.D. diss., Boston College 1983.

Leighow, Susan Rimby. "Backrubs vs. Bach: Nursing and the Entry-into-Practice Debate." Paper presented at the History of Education Society Annual Meeting, Atlanta, Ga., November 3, 1990.

Index

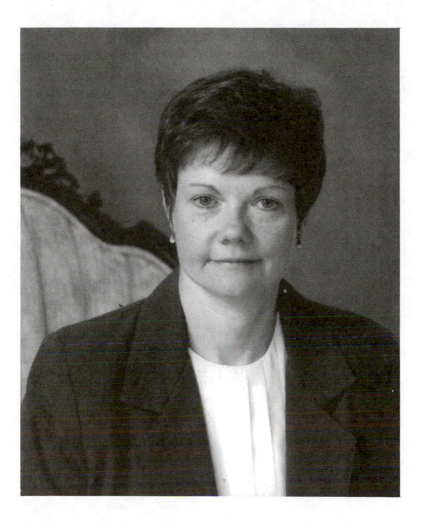

Susan Rimby Leighow is an assistant professor of History at Shippensburg University of Pennsylvania. She received her Ph.D. in United States History from the University of Pittsburgh. She has published several articles in journals and anthologies.